Basics of
Computer Vision Syndrome

Basics of Computer Vision Syndrome

Second Edition

Ajay Kumar Bhootra
B Optom DOS FAO FOAI FCLI
ICLEP FIACLE (Australia)
Diploma in Sportvision (UK)
Ex-CEO and Dean
Krishnalaya School of Optometry
Kolkata, West Bengal, India

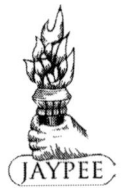

JAYPEE BROTHERS MEDICAL PUBLISHERS
The Health Sciences Publisher
New Delhi | London

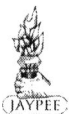 **Jaypee Brothers Medical Publishers (P) Ltd.**

Headquarters
Jaypee Brothers Medical Publishers (P) Ltd.
EMCA House, 23/23-B
Ansari Road, Daryaganj
New Delhi 110 002, India
Landline: +91-11-23272143, +91-11-23272703
+91-11-23282021, +91-11-23245672
Email: jaypee@jaypeebrothers.com

Corporate Office
Jaypee Brothers Medical Publishers (P) Ltd.
4838/24, Ansari Road, Daryaganj
New Delhi 110 002, India
Phone: +91-11-43574357
Fax: +91-11-43574314
Email: jaypee@jaypeebrothers.com

Overseas Office
J.P. Medical Ltd.
83 Victoria Street, London
SW1H 0HW (UK)
Phone: +44 20 3170 8910
Fax: +44 (0)20 3008 6180
Email: info@jpmedpub.com

Website: www.jaypeebrothers.com
Website: www.jaypeedigital.com

© 2023, Jaypee Brothers Medical Publishers

The views and opinions expressed in this book are solely those of the original contributor(s)/author(s) and do not necessarily represent those of editor(s) and publisher of the book.

All rights reserved. No part of this publication may be reproduced, stored or transmitted in any form or by any means, electronic, mechanical, photocopying, recording or otherwise, without the prior permission in writing of the publishers.

All brand names and product names used in this book are trade names, service marks, trademarks or registered trademarks of their respective owners. The publisher is not associated with any product or vendor mentioned in this book.

Medical knowledge and practice change constantly. This book is designed to provide accurate, authoritative information about the subject matter in question. However, readers are advised to check the most current information available on procedures included and check information from the manufacturer of each product to be administered, to verify the recommended dose, formula, method and duration of administration, adverse effects and contraindications. It is the responsibility of the practitioner to take all appropriate safety precautions. Neither the publisher nor the author(s)/editor(s) assume any liability for any injury and/or damage to persons or property arising from or related to use of material in this book.

This book is sold on the understanding that the publisher is not engaged in providing professional medical services. If such advice or services are required, the services of a competent medical professional should be sought.

Every effort has been made where necessary to contact holders of copyright to obtain permission to reproduce copyright material. If any have been inadvertently overlooked, the publisher will be pleased to make the necessary arrangements at the first opportunity.

Inquiries for bulk sales may be solicited at: jaypee@jaypeebrothers.com

Basics of Computer Vision Syndrome

First Edition: 2014

Second Edition: **2023**

ISBN: 978-93-5696-176-0

Printed at India

Dedicated to
All members of my family

Preface to the Second Edition

The introduction of computers and advancements in technology have not only revolutionized and benefited society but also given rise to new ocular, visual, and muscular difficulties caused by interaction with computer screens and their environments. Visual stress, irritation, redness, dryness, blurred vision, and double vision are common symptoms among most computer users. These symptoms taken together are known as "Computer Vision Syndrome." Three mechanisms that led to computer vision syndrome are extraocular functions, accommodative functions, and ocular surface anomalies.

While the society was struggling to create the awareness among the computer users for protection of eyes from computer use, the new advancement in technology during the last decade has completely changed the lifestyle of almost everyone in the society. Several influencing digital gadgets were added to human life, and we started using them from the time we get up in the morning until the time we go to bed again, including the time when we are eating, exercising, working, relaxing, communicating, and reading, when we are using one or another digital device. Often, we use them simultaneously instead of sequentially. In fact, we cannot seem to live without them.

The impact has been seen in changing the visual postures and behavior patterns of users. The main effect of prolonged exposure to these light-emitting devices is being noticed as "digital eye strain," which manifests itself in different ways with symptoms like red eyes, dry eyes, irritated eyes, neck pain, and shoulder pain. Our multi-screen lifestyle is a direct cause of discomfort and dysfunction.

These new developments forced researchers to relook at the symptoms of "Computer Vision Syndrome," as they were very similar to what they noticed with digital gadget users, and they started referring to "Computer Vision Syndrome" (CVS) as "Digital Vision Syndrome" (DVS). DVS symptoms are the same as CVS symptoms like eye strain, headache, blurred vision, etc. These can be seen in literally any age group.

Digital eye strain is more real than reality now. The truth is, people are not going to stop using these digital devices. The industry has responded to these changes by providing new categories of lenses for a connected life. As professionals, optometrists have to figure out how to extend their services because people are not going to stop using these digital devices. Sometimes the simplest solution is the one most often overlooked. There has to be a continuous focus on it, both in terms of professional care and appropriate treatment management. It is a known fact that early intervention reduces the prevalence of visual discomfort among digital gadget users. This is where this book will fit in the most.

This book is an effort aimed at providing resource materials to those who would like to establish their practice as "Computer Vision Specialists." Although the author does not claim it to be a comprehensive book, it is good enough to kick things off. More research and studies would definitely be needed. Hence, readers are strongly encouraged to keep themselves updated with the help of other resources as well. Students will be highly benefitted because the book is very simple and precise with relevant multiple choice questions and also questions for their self practice.

I wish you a good read and the very best in your journey towards becoming a successful "Computer Vision Specialist."

Ajay Kumar Bhootra

Preface to the First Edition

The introduction of computers during 1970 gave rise to lot of stormy controversial debate. The controversy was wide-ranging from workplace ergonomics, lighting to health and work stress. Soon, it was detected that computer operator reported some common visual symptoms that were not so commonly seen before, which fuelled the fears that computers may harm vision. This provided a new platform for the researchers, especially about the claims that intensive visual work with computer screens will damage the eyes. However, computers are now accepted as an integral part of life; we use them at work and at home and also while leisure without so much second thought. Computers are no more special. In fact, the application of computers has totally transformed the lifestyle of the human being, restricting the movement of body as well as limiting the viewing range. The problem is not only limited to adults. Many children use computers for educational and recreational purposes. The way the children use the computers may make them even more susceptible to the development of computer-related vision symptoms. Children often continue performing their enjoyable task without breaks until they are near exhaustion. Such prolonged activity may increase eye-focusing problems and eye irritation. An additional issue is that computer workstations are typically arranged for adults. Therefore, a child using computer on such typical arrangement may result in one or more computer-related vision symptoms.

This calls into question the term "Computer Vision Syndrome"— A widely spreading but largely unknown epidemic among computer users. Today computer-related eyestrain is considered as the No. 1 office health complaint in the world. Despite the large number of people are affected by computer-related problems—many of them have not heard of computer vision syndrome. This may be considered as an alarming condition for India where health consciousness is still far behind.

It is a known fact that early intervention reduces the prevalence of visual discomfort among computer users. There is no question that employers have an increased obligation to ensure that workplace and work tasks are well-designed and do not impose unnecessary physical and psychological stress. It is also their duty that they should arrange regular eye check up for their employees. Ophthalmologists and optometrists should also assure that any individual working for more than two hours at a stretch on computers should be given specialized eye care services. School teachers should also talk about computer vision syndrome while lecturing on various aspects of computer science. Parents must ensure that their children should have periodic eye examination with necessary treatment. In fact, we all need to remember that:

"*An ounce of prevention is worth a pound of cure.*"

Ajay Kumar Bhootra

Acknowledgments

As far as I understand, no creation in this world is a solo effort, neither is this book. I have received enormous inputs from several people, from the time I conceived the idea of this book to its present shape. I would like to acknowledge everybody's efforts and would like to thank all of them for bringing it to this shape.

A special thanks to:
- My students for their love and affection,
- God, Who cares for me,
- My family, who always bear with semblance of smile seeing me engaged in writing day in and day out,
- My amazing list of patients and clients because of whom I could have such varied experiences,
- All my trainers and coaches whose training sessions I have attended,
- My friends and well-wishers,
- And all those people who have helped me understand my subjects,
- And above all, the members of my organization - Himalaya Optical.

Finally, I would like to acknowledge the power of motivation that I get from Albert Einstein's quote when he said, **'I have no special talents. I am only passionately curious'**.

Contents

1. **Computer and Vision** 1
   - Vision and Visual System 2
   - Visual Demands for Computer Work 4
   - Computer and Body Posture 8
   - Computer and Blink Rate 10

2. **Computer Vision Syndrome** 13
   - Visual Symptoms 13
   - Ocular Symptoms 15
   - Asthenopic Symptoms 16
   - Light Sensitivity Symptoms 17
   - Musculoskeletal Symptoms 18
   - General Symptoms 20

3. **Laws of Computer Vision** 23

4. **Understanding Patient, Patient's Visual Environment, and Visual System** 31
   - History-taking 32
   - Visual Acuity Test 35
   - Dominant Eye Test 36
   - Objective Assessment of Eye 38

5. **Correction of Refractive Error for Computer Vision Syndrome Patient** 43
   - Symptoms 43
   - Rationale 43
   - Types of Refractive Error 44
   - Cycloplegic Refraction 45
   - Refractive Error Correction 46

6. **Accommodative Function and its Management** 52
   - Symptoms 52
   - Rationale 52
   - Accommodative Function 53
   - Clinical Examination of Accommodation Function 56
   - Treatment 61

7. **Binocular Vision and its Management** 63
   - Symptoms *63*
   - Rationale *63*
   - Two Eyes—As a Pair *64*
   - Clinical Examination of Binocular Vision *66*
   - Treatment *72*

8. **Eye Movement Disorder and its Management** 75
   - Symptoms *75*
   - Rationale *75*
   - Important Eye Movement Skills for Reading *77*
   - Clinical Examination of Ocular Motor Dysfunction *79*
   - Treatment *80*

9. **Computer Use and Dry Eye** 82
   - Symptoms *82*
   - Rationale *82*
   - Diagnosis of Dry Eyes *85*
   - Management *88*

10. **Issues Related to Glare and Reflection** 91
    - Glare *91*
    - Reflection *96*
    - Role of Antireflection Coated Lenses *98*
    - Role of Blue Cut Lenses *100*

11. **Presbyopia and Computer Use** 105
    - Symptoms *105*
    - Rationale *105*
    - Diagnosis of Presbyopia *106*
    - Computer and Presbyopia *111*

12. **Computer-workstation Arrangement** 119
    - Issues Related to Body Posture *120*
    - Issues Related to Furniture and Fixture *122*
    - Issues Related to Hardware and Attachment *125*
    - Issues Related to Computer Display *126*
    - Ideal Sitting Posture While Working on a Computer *128*
    - Ideal Computer Workstation *129*

13. **Sequential Management Considerations** 131
    - Initial Management *131*
    - Subsequent Follow Ups *132*
    - Ergonomic Issues *134*
14. **Building up the Practice as a CVS Specialist** 136
    - Getting Started *138*
    - Place Planning to Set Up the Practice *140*
    - Setting Up the Practice *140*
    - Promotions and Marketing *141*
    - Practice Management *146*
    - Stand Proud and have Self-commitment *147*
15. **Vision Screening Program for Computer Users** 149
    - Battery of Vision Screen Tests *151*

Appendix *157*
Bibliography *159*
Index *161*

CHAPTER 1

Computer and Vision

In ancient times, when human beings used to live in forests, their primary occupation was hunting and the primary visual need was to look at distance to hunt in an effort to arrange the food for their life. With civilization, there had been enormous changes in the lifestyle. Suddenly, they found themselves confined to their tables and chairs working on computers and spending most of their time within a small boundary of offices. The change also had its effect on the primary visual demands. The "distance-dominant world" suddenly changed to complete "near-point world". Most tasks, whether on job or otherwise, shifted to near-point distance or intermediate distance **(Fig. 1.1)**. The increased confinement to near-point world has its own effect on our vision and visual system. There is a basic difference between seeing more at near and seeing more at distance. Near-point vision implies that:

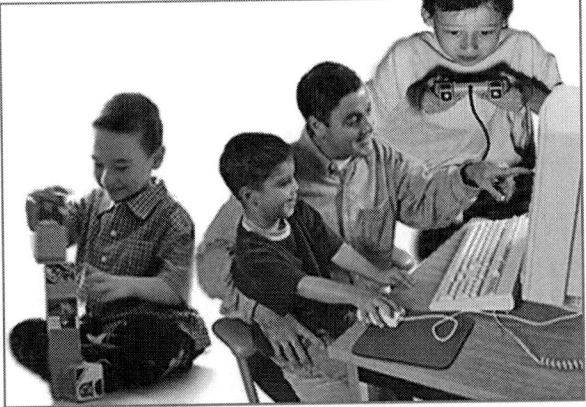

Fig. 1.1: Near-point world.

- There is constant stress upon the accommodative system of human eyes.
- Convergence functions of the eyes are also active.

The straightforward meaning is that 6/6 or 20/20 at distance is no more the conclusive evidence of a healthy visual system.

The impact was noticed as an adverse effect on most elements of visual system that produced both temporary and permanent adaptive changes which include:
- Nearsightedness
- Suppressed vision in one eye
- Poor eye teaming
- Reduced performance both at work and at play.

This is an important issue as far as occupational performance of the computer workers is concerned as occupational performance depends upon the visual performance. But, it is a more serious issue for the development of children as they are very susceptible. A child who is addicted to computer may develop fast eyes and good brain, but his general physical health may be mess. The computer games are one step ahead in harming. The fight-and-flight situation during computer games increases the secretion of the cholesterol and adrenalin and provide no physical relaxation. This is a recipe for the early grave. Many people may not be able to handle the visual stress of prolonged near work and simply cannot deal with computer-related visual stress, resulting in many direct and indirect symptoms which can be grouped under computer vision syndrome or CVS.

VISION AND VISUAL SYSTEM

Vision may be defined as an act of seeing. It may be with contact lenses or with spectacle or may be without any optical aid. It can be maximized by the correct use of lenses and the right choice of tints. Vision is the ability to take in the information through the eyes and derive meaning from it. It implies taking the information and initiating the appropriate response. The two eyes capture the image and transmit to the brain where the two images are fused together, interpreted and integrated as a three-dimensional phenomenon. The brain then sends the message as electric signals, down to the spinal cords to the arms or leg muscles telling them to move. The whole process is preprogramed automatic so that minimum attention is required for information acquisition and processing.

Good vision provides spatial awareness and efficient discriminating ability. It also involves the ability to use the eyes for an extended period of time without discomfort, to analyze and interpret information and to respond to what is being seen. Good vision allows an individual to perform the visual task seamlessly at any point of time of the day, regardless of the task or environment.

Vision is the complex process. Multiple components work together under a feedback loop to gather, focus, capture, and process light to make sense out of vision. Visual acuity is the fundamental characteristic of the visual system and is the prime determinant of any regimen that aims to improve visual and occupational performance. Visual acuity defines the acuteness or sharpness of vision, i.e., the ability to perceive the fine details. It is the spatial resolving capacity of the visual system. It expresses the angular size of the object that can be just resolved by the observer. It can also be defined as the time-dependent measurement of retinal health. 6/6 or 20/20 measured on Snellen's chart denotes optimum visual acuity. But visual acuity alone cannot tell us anything about the reasons for headache after reading, intermittent blurring of text, loss of place while reading, seeing double while reading, and many more such conditions. These problems are also associated with visual system that affects visual performance. There are other elements of visual system— they are accommodation, binocular vision system, and eye movements. Accommodation is basically focusing mechanism that occurs as reflex action when focus changes from distance to near and vice versa. Binocular vision system allows two eyes to work as a team to provide sustained comfortable and clear single vision. The oculomotor system controls and coordinates the movements of two eyes while tracking the object. The ocular motor system directs and holds both eyes on to the object. With two eyes working together as a team, there are so many visual skills needed for single and clear vision for a sustained period of time. Excess of visual demands on any of the skills of visual system leads to symptoms. When an individual is working on the computer, his eyes are converged, i.e., turn inward toward the nose and there is a constant stress on his ocular accommodation. Constant stress on convergence and accommodation function questions the abilities of these functions. The situation is worsened by the limitations of office ergonomics coupled with glare and reflection of light and screen to create a situation where the operator reports the visual symptoms due to visual problems related to computer use.

VISUAL DEMANDS FOR COMPUTER WORK

Most eye care professionals agree that computer users demonstrate unique eye and vision problems, and the sources for such problems are not only individual visual system but also the ergonomics of the work environment. The list of change starts with the difference in letter types with which they need to work. The letter types that are printed with solid black color on a white background paper show well-defined edges with good contrast between its background and the letters. On the other hand, electronically generated letter types that are displayed on computer screens are made of small dots or pixels. These pixilated letters have poorly defined edges. They are brightest in the center and diminish in contrast at the edges **(Fig. 1.2)**. Human eyes and brain react very well to the most printed materials that have good contrast, whereas they react differently to those pixelated characters. They are optically imperfect characters, and sometimes even the perfectly functioning eyes have difficulties maintaining accurate focus on such imperfect characters.

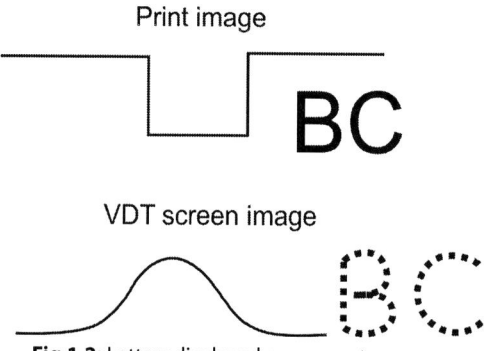

Fig.1.2: Letters displayed on computer screen.

The second major difference is because of the illuminated letters and the background. The light emitted by the computer monitor when it interacts with the lights of visual environment causes glare in the visual field. Glare creates veiling effect and reduces contrast. It also adds to the visual stress. The result is noticed in the form of reduced ability to sustain the focus on the plane of computer screen.

Another important difference is the viewing distance at which they work. The computer monitor is usually placed at a distance of 50–60 cm which is slightly more than the usual reading distance and significantly less than the long viewing distance. It means that the accommodative mechanism of the visual system is always active. Besides, different occupations on computer have different visual demands. Those who are primarily on computer designing or net surfing or any other job that needs constant viewing on screen demonstrate different visual demands than those who are mostly engaged in data feeding from a source document to the system. Each occupational need on computer has to be evaluated separately before deciding upon the management. The change in viewing angle while working on a computer monitor also has its own effect. Moreover, most computer-related tasks are repetitive and can become stressful both mentally and physically after an extended period of continuous work. The eyes end up being overworked, and this can result in eyestrain.

In such a highly visually demanding task where there is always a possibility that the visual demands for an individual concerned may exceed his visual ability, it is very critical to look at eyes and the visual system as a total system where each element may contribute to symptoms. The common elements of the visual system that must be addressed are as follows:
- Visual acuity
- Contrast
- Accommodative system
- Binocular vision
- Oculomotor skills
- Depth perception
- Color perception

1. **Visual acuity:** More than 90% information received is through the vision. Good vision is the most important attribute that

involves the ability to use the eyes for an extended period of time without any discomfort. Vision is the function of visual acuity. It can be improved by optimizing the visual acuity in a clinical setup with a specific test chart placed at a specific test distance. Good refraction is the primary requirement in achieving the optimal visual acuity. Unless visual acuity is maximized during the refraction, all other aspects of eye examination have no meaning. This becomes more critical when there is a pressure of excess visual demands on the visual system. Traditional eye examination for near vision is for reading distance at 40 cm, but most computer screens are placed at a distance which is always more than normal reading distance. Besides, printed texts are used for near-vision eye examination, not the pixelated text of computer monitors. Our eyes react differently to the stimulus of computer letters. Therefore, improving visual acuity at the specific computer monitor distance with computer-simulated targets is very critical for improving visual acuity for computer tasks. An improved acuity will aid to aiming and focusing at the computer monitor for comfortable working. Uncorrected or under corrected refractive error can be major contributing factors to computer-related eye stress. Sometimes, even a small amount of astigmatism can also result in symptoms because of acuity demands of the task. This would translate to loss of an employee's productivity because of increase in the employee's fatigue. The problem becomes more critical in presbyopia when the normal glasses that meet their visual needs for most other tasks usually do not properly correct their vision for computer display.

2. **Contrast:** Good contrast makes characters more legible. Contrast is typically limited by the darkness of "black" on the display. Better contrast is attained with darker black. Contrast is the function of corrected visual acuity. It is also affected because of media opacities that result in light scattering. Reflection from the display and glare in the visual environment also result in the reduced contrast of text presented on the screen. The decreased contrast makes it more difficult for the eyes to fixate and focus, maintain binocularity, and move over the text quickly and efficiently. Working under these conditions increases the demand on the visual system.

3. **Accommodative system:** Most computer tasks are either at near or extended near-viewing distance. The computer workers have to accommodate to look at the keyboard and then to look up at the screen, again to the written text and back to the screen. It implies that the visual system is always in a state of accommodative stress. This cycle continues for several hours. Allowance for efficient accommodative system is therefore very critical to prolonged comfortable computer viewing. An improper functioning of the accommodative system is normally the cause of intermittent blurring of near objects, such as the computer screen or reference document, and is also responsible for temporary blurring of distance objects after working at near distance for an extended period of time.
4. **Binocular vision:** The very nature of most computer tasks implies that the person is either looking at near or extended near-viewing distance. Eye alignment at near-viewing distance is more complex than at distance because of ocular convergence required to view near objects. Convergence is also associated with accommodation. Poor convergence ability in computer users result in symptoms of eyestrain and eye fatigue. Convergence insufficiency is quite common in the population as a whole.

    However, people who do not perform a demanding visual task may not develop symptoms from it. But in symptomatic subjects, it is quite likely that even a small amount of vertical or horizontal phorias need to be corrected to ease the symptoms.
5. **Oculomotor skills:** It is controlled by extraocular muscles outside the eye and networked with the brain. It is an important skill to maintain binocular vision. It is the ability of moving our eyes quickly and accurately so that we can direct and maintain a steady fixation on an object of regard. The two oculomotor skills are very important, i.e., saccades and pursuits. Saccade moves the eyes from one point to another point as it is observed while reading, whereas pursuit is efficient tracking of a moving object. Regression is another important oculomotor skill for reading. It is a backward movement of the eye when reading a line of text. The function of these "regressions" is still largely unknown. The most acceptable explanation is that regressions allow for the rereading of previously fixated words, effectively aiding the comprehension process.

6. **Depth perception:** Depth perception or stereoacuity is an important aspect of normal and healthy vision. It is being considered as the barometer of binocular vision. The quality of binocular vision is higher with finer stereoacuity. Any anomalies in the stereoacuity suggest that the binocular vision system is not working efficiently or, in other words, suppression and excessive fixation disparity may lead to reduction in stereoacuity. Stereoacuity is more critical at close viewing distance than far distance. The computer worker works predominantly at close viewing distance. Good stereoacuity is needed to see the figures in their three-dimensional structures, locate the relative position of the supplementary hardware and materials for smooth functioning, and also follow the text on the screen and source document.
7. **Color perception:** It is a very important consideration while developing websites and other designing tasks. Missing color information can be as much of a problem as missing words in written text. If a color is a primary carrier of information and is confused or not seen, transfer of information is reduced. Color vision may be altered because of many reasons. Color vision defect may be inherited or may be acquired. Sometimes, it may alter because of drugs, medications, or toxic effects of chemicals. The status of color vision examination forms an important part of the overall eye examination and it may also help in differential diagnosis.

COMPUTER AND BODY POSTURE

Natural posture while working for a day-long activity is very important to minimize the undue strain on the body. The straightforward meaning is that the working station has to be designed considering the human factor. In essence, the human factor implies that all furniture, equipment, and other devices should be designed to fit the human body and its cognitive abilities. The workstation so designed will allow natural posture and will not force to adapt any uncomfortable postures such as hunching over, slouching, straining, or twisting **(Fig. 1.3)**. Working for extended lengths of time in an ergonomically designed workstation will not result in any musculoskeletal issues.

Chapter 1: Computer and Vision

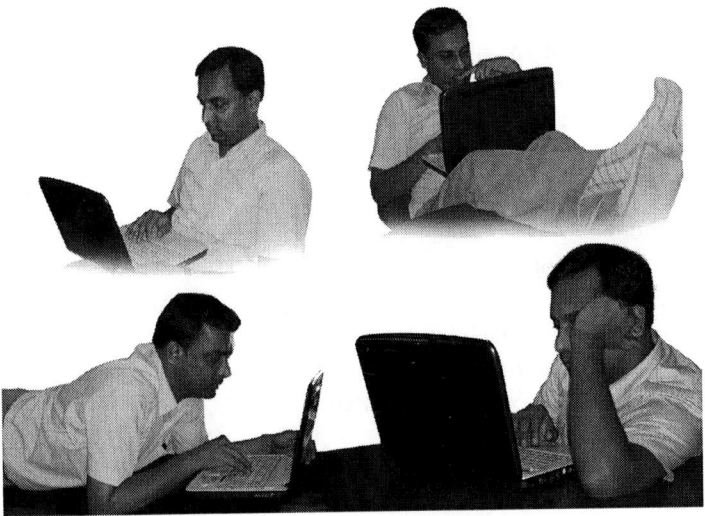

Fig.1.3: Incorrect body postures.

The difficulties with workstation may include the following:
- Using a chair that is of wrong height or size
- Using a chair that does not support the back
- Using a chair that does not support the hand
- Incorrect height of work surfaces like desktop and keyboard
- Inadequate space between chair and working table, not allowing any body movement
- Improper lighting arrangements creating sources of glare in the visual field.

The location of the visual target plays a major role in determining sitting posture. In an effort to position the body so that the face is parallel to the viewing plane, the person assumes unusual posture which may cause poor posture and thereby neck pain, back pain, and also carpal tunnel. Therefore, the placement of a computer monitor plays an important role in designing the computer workstation. In general, the top of the monitor should come to approximately your mid-forehead when it is adjusted to the proper height. However, the monitor positioning has to be altered for a bifocal lens user.

Another important fact that has to be kept in mind is that the human body is not designed to sit still for a long period of time even in correct position. Depending upon the work and environment, you may want to take breaks. Even while sitting, you may feel like stretching and relaxing your body. The basic stretching can work wonderfully to warm you up again in preparation to continue the work for an extended period of time.

Thus, the location and position of monitor together with ergonomically designed furniture determine sitting posture and visual angles of the computer worker so that he can help himself to naturally align in a more efficient and beneficial way for maximum comfort and stamina at the workplace. This is also important to enhance the productivity of the employee as an uncomfortable employee will eventually become less productive.

COMPUTER AND BLINK RATE

Blinking **(Fig. 1.4)** helps spread tears across and removes irritants from the surface of the cornea and conjunctiva. Blink rate represents the frequency of blink recorded over a specific time period. Blink rate may be influenced by many elements. A normal individual in normal circumstances blinks approximately 15 times per minute which may

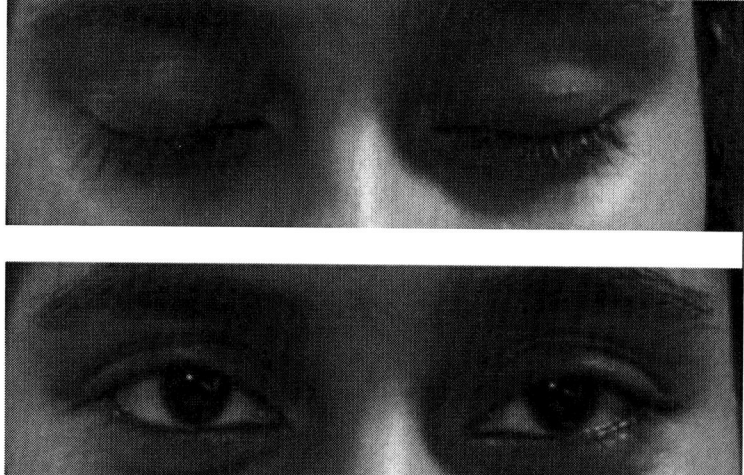

Fig.1.4: Blinking.

be increased to 21-23 blinks per minute during relaxed condition and may be reduced to 7 blinks per minute while viewing text on computer display and 4 blinks per minute during extensive computer use. The reason for decreased rate of blink may be attributed to concentration needed for computer task and/or a relatively limited range of eye movement. Although book reading and other intensive near tasks also result in significantly decreased blink rates, computer work usually requires a higher gaze angle, resulting in most incomplete blinks. Incomplete blink is like no blink. Reduced blink rate coupled with a larger size of the ocular aperture is the primary cause of tear elimination through evaporation which makes them experience ocular drying and foreign body sensation.

Multiple Choice Questions-Answers

1. **What is considered to be normal blink rate?**
   a. 6 blinks/minute
   b. 12 blinks/minute
   c. 15 blinks/minute
   d. 8 blinks/minute

2. **Which of the following visual skills is often termed the barometer of the binocular vision?**
   a. Accommodation
   b. Stereoacuity
   c. Convergence
   d. Color perception

3. **Which of the following is not the part of near-vision trio?**
   a. Accommodation is active
   b. Accommodation is relaxed
   c. Two eyes converge
   d. Pupil constricts

Answer Key

| 1. | (c) | 2. | (b) | 3. | (b) |

Self-Practice Questions

1. Explain the meaning of the term "Computer Vision Syndrome".
2. Explain the influence of computer use on blink rate.
3. Why does body posture and body position matter while working on computer?

CHAPTER 2

Computer Vision Syndrome

Computer vision syndrome (CVS) by itself is not denoting any condition; instead, it includes all those numerous symptoms that are eye and vision related and are associated with the computer use. It also includes some of the musculoskeletal problems that may arise because of computer-working environment. CVS is a temporary condition and commonly arises because visual demands of the occupation exceed the visual ability of the person concerned. The condition is further aggravated by the improper lighting condition or workplace-surrounding environments. Most people who spend long hours looking at a computer monitor, whether it be for work, play, or a combination of the two, are most likely to present the symptoms of CVS. The various symptoms of CVS may be grouped in **Flowchart 2.1**.

VISUAL SYMPTOMS

Most of the visual symptoms of the computer worker are related to the blurred vision and symptoms arising because of blurred vision. They complain that they find it difficult to maintain clear and steady focus for a significant amount of time, and sometimes refocusing is slow. Often, they find themselves lost while reading text documents. Squinting the eyes enables them to read clearly. All of these symptoms

Flowchart 2.1: Symptoms of CVS.

```
                    CVS
  ┌──────┬──────┬──────┬──────┬──────┬──────┐
Visual  Ocular  Asthenopic  Light   Musculo-  General
symptoms symptoms         sensitivity skeletal
```

usually point to the presence of refractive error. Blurred vision (**Fig. 2.1**) may be of different types:
- Constant blurred vision
- Postwork distance blur
- Intermittent blurred vision at near.

1. Constant blurred vision is an indication of an uncorrected or undercorrected myopia, hypermetropia, astigmatism, or presbyopia, depending upon the viewing distance at which the blur occurs. The person complaining of blurred vision often squints his eyes to overcome the symptoms.
2. Delay in focusing at distance after working for a long period of time for near work is mostly the characteristic feature of an accommodation being locked at near-viewing distance or general accommodative dysfunction. This kind of blurred vision may be momentary when the person looks up from his near work or may last for several hours after near work.
3. Intermittent blurred vision at near-viewing distance may also be caused by dry eyes. A careful history taking by asking the patient whether his vision clears just after he blinks may help diagnose it.

In extreme cases, symptoms related to double vision may be reported which straightaway points toward binocular vision dysfunction. It often gets worse as the day passes or reading extends beyond a few minutes. However, people complaining of double vision are so sensitive that they either close their one eye or try to change

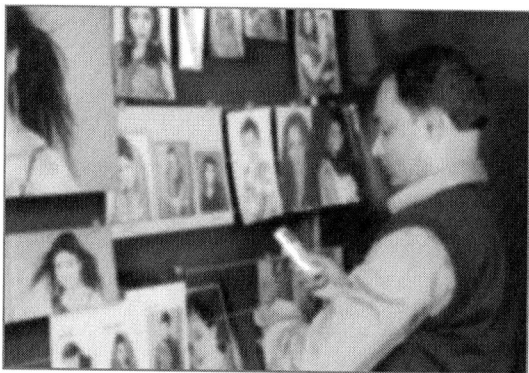

Fig. 2.1: Blurred vision.

their visual posture to overcome it. The occasional color perception problems may be because of poor display quality of the screen. Poor contrast and the presence of glare may also affect color perception temporarily.

OCULAR SYMPTOMS

Poor blinking rate, incomplete blinking, horizontal visual gaze, and wide-open palpebral aperture during computer tasks lead to dry and irritated eyes. The person often complains of itching eyes (**Fig. 2.2**), burning eyes, foreign body sensation, and/or sore eyes (**Fig. 2.3**). At times, the condition manifests in the form of excessive tears and

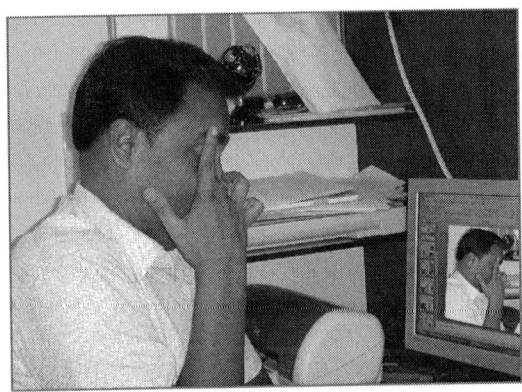

Fig. 2.2: Itching eyes.

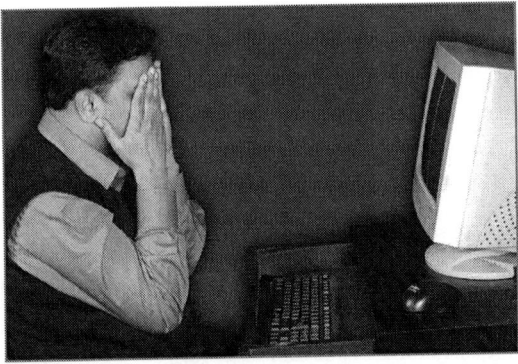

Fig. 2.3: Sore eyes.

excessive blinks. Wide-open eyes with horizontal visual gaze angle at the screen cause tear evaporation that results in loss of tears. The condition aggravates because of low humidity of the office air that also adds to dryness. Dry eyes result in reflex tears and foreign body sensation. A complaint of watery eyes is often the result of reflex tearing secondary to irritation caused by dry eyes. Irritated or burning eyes in the absence of dry eyes may indicate the presence of toxic elements in the office atmosphere which may be confirmed if the other employees also have similar symptoms.

ASTHENOPIC SYMPTOMS

Asthenopia is more commonly known as eyestrain or visual fatigue. It is a common condition that occurs when the eyes become tired from intense use. The manifestation of eyestrain is because of the following reasons:
- Extreme visual demands of computer use
- Inefficiency of the visual system
- General health that determines the ability of an individual to withstand the sustained effort.

Staring at a computer screen for a long period of time is overtaxing of the ciliary muscles and to this is added strain of the neuromuscular control of the ocular movements in order to maintain convergence and compensate for heterophoria, if present. Illumination is the principal environmental factor responsible for eyestrain. The person complaining eyestrain often reports that he feels more comfortable when the illumination level is reduced. The condition may be aggravated because of poor ergonomics such as glare and reflection around the working environment. The ocular factors that cause eye strain are uncorrected ametropia, accommodation difficulties, convergence difficulties, heterophoria, fusional inadequacies, and aniseikonia. The general health of the computer user is also sometimes the reason that determines eyestrain as the break point is more readily reached in a feeble than in a robust individual.

The visual fatigue, associated with ocular pain for a computer user, is mostly muscular in nature. It is usually mild and dull for a computer user. Constantly altering levels of ciliary and extraocular muscular activities may be the fatiguing factor.

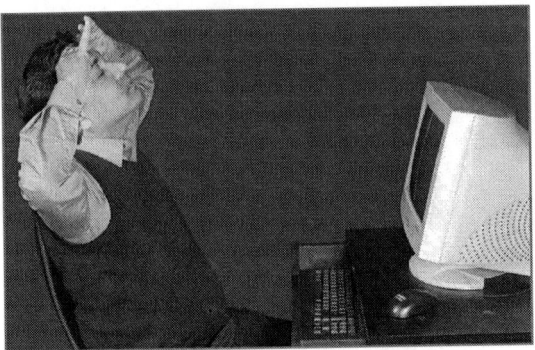

Fig. 2.4: Headache.

Headache (**Fig. 2.4**) is the most common symptom associated with eyestrain. Visual headaches most often occur toward the front of the head, of course with some exceptions, occur most often toward the middle or end of the day, do not appear upon awakening, often occur in a different pattern on weekends than during the week, or can occur on one side of the head more than the other. These can be precipitated by many forms of stress, including anxiety and depression, numerous eye conditions, and improper workplace conditions. In some cases, a binocular vision disorder may also result in light sensitivity and glaring effect. The sensitivity of glare is amplified as light scatters in the optical medium of the eyes. Trying to read a degraded image can certainly contribute to eyestrain or other visual discomfort. This may make focusing a stressful task difficult, which may cause headache and other disturbances.

It must be remembered that the gross visual errors do not give rise to typical symptoms of eyestrain. It is the small error that the subject can rectify to some extent or to a greater extent by muscular effort, which is the main reason for eyestrain. The straightforward understanding is that it is not the error itself that causes the trouble so much as the continuous effort in an attempt to correct the same, initiated automatically.

LIGHT SENSITIVITY SYMPTOMS

Light sensitivity can result from several conditions. The following conditions can be noticed while working on computers:

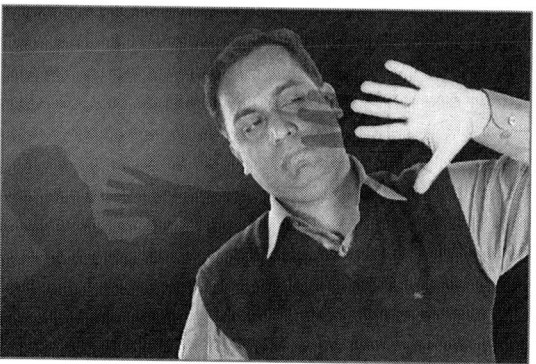

Fig. 2.5: Effect of glare.

- The horizontal gaze angle that is quite commonly seen during a computer task is always higher than the gaze angle needed for reading or other table tasks. The result is bright light sources of the office which are closer to central fixation.
- The computer worker is constantly gazing at the illuminated target, which is absolutely in contrast with reading printed targets.
- Glare (**Fig. 2.5**) and reflections are present in the office atmosphere due to fluorescent light or reflections because of screen and other surfaces may create light pollution in and around the computer working station.

Moreover, in some cases, a binocular vision disorder may also result in light sensitivity. The person may report flickering sensation and light sensitivity. In extreme cases, the patient may report pain in the eyes.

MUSCULOSKELETAL SYMPTOMS

The typical posture of the computer worker while working on the computer can be explained as under:

"He sits on a chair that fits to his body size or slightly larger, keeps his wrists on the keyboard with the elbow at an angle between the keyboard top and the chair handle top, neck upright with eyes gazing straight ahead on the display monitor with overall stiff body posture. The working station does not allow for much body movement and he maintains similar postures for hours together."

The human body is not suitable to work for an extended period of time in the same posture. Experience has shown that an individual who maintains the same posture for a longer period of time most commonly reports:
- Neck aches **(Fig. 2.6)**
- Shoulder pain
- Backaches
- Wrist pain **(Fig. 2.7)**
- Pain in arms
- Pain in waist **(Fig. 2.8)**

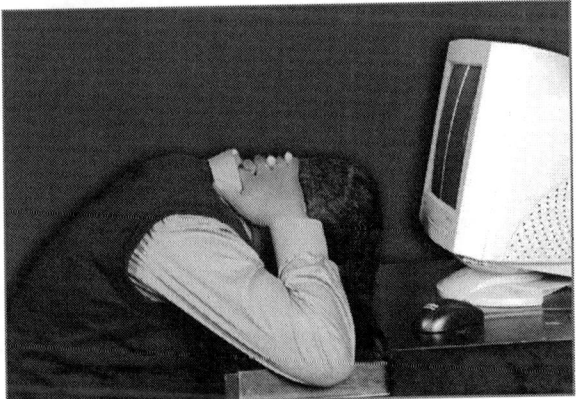

Fig. 2.6: Neck ache.

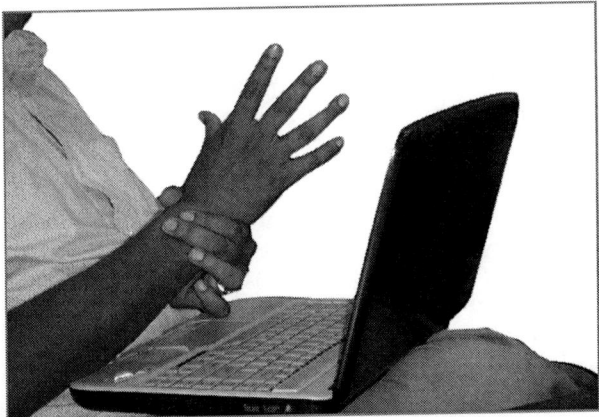

Fig. 2.7: Wrist pain.

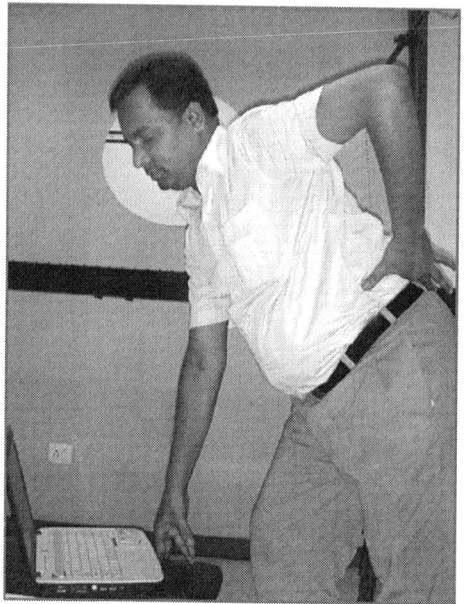

Fig. 2.8: Pain in waist.

This is not only common with computer users but also with other workers engaged in repetitive work. These musculoskeletal symptoms result from inadequate body movement and undesirable posture for an extended period of time, which creates stress on body muscles. The position of wrists and hands on keyboard is the cause of pain in arms and wrists. Carpal tunnel syndrome is quite often seen in a computer user. In many office situations, the vision of a worker is compromised and he must adapt his posture to ease the strain on the visual system. These situations may cause obvious physical problems that can be easily remedied with the proper lenses.

GENERAL SYMPTOMS

General symptoms such as tension, physical fatigue, irritability, increased nervousness, frequent error, general fatigue, and drowsiness are usually the cumulative effect of multiple factors. The stress involved in repetitive computer task, stiff body postures because of working station, coupled with pressure of targets to finish job in time

Chapter 2: Computer Vision Syndrome

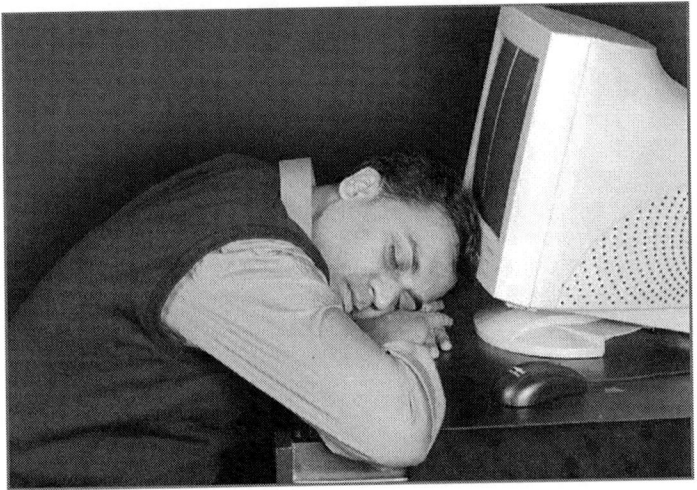

Fig. 2.9: General fatigue.

by itself are enough to create tensions, physical fatigue, nervousness, and irritability. When they are compounded by the personal problems also, the effect is manifested in the form of headache, drowsiness, and general fatigue **(Fig. 2.9)**. These symptoms are not directly linked to eyes, but it is always like one factor becomes the reason for another and vice versa. Visual headache most often occurs toward the mid or end of the day. It does not appear early in the morning. At times, other ocular symptoms and visual and musculoskeletal symptoms add to general fatigue. If all obvious factors are looked at, medical management may often start with a complete eye examination.

Multiple Choice Questions-Answers

1. **Symptoms associated with CVS can largely be categorized into one of the following areas:**
   a. Refractive error and binocular vision disorder
   b. Ocular surface health
   c. Ergonomics
   d. All of the above

2. CVS is a group of eye and vision-related problems resulting from an extended period of computer use. Which of the following symptoms is associated with CVS?
   a. Eyestrain and headache
   b. Dry eyes
   c. Neck and shoulder pain
   d. All of the above

3. Which of the following is not the ocular factor responsible for eye strain while working on a computer?
   a. Uncorrected ametropia
   b. Aniseikonia
   c. Illumination
   d. Heterophoria

Answer Key

| 1. | (d) | 2. | (d) | 3. | (c) |

Self-Practice Questions

1. "Computer vision syndrome by itself does not denote any condition; instead, it is a group of symptoms that are associated with VDU use." What are they? Explain.

2. "The gross visual error does not give rise to symptoms of eyestrain; instead, it is the small error in any of the visual skills that causes symptoms of eyestrain." Explain with examples how it may happen for an intense computer user.

CHAPTER 3

Laws of Computer Vision

The increasing applications of the computer in the last few decades have great influence on our visual system. It is absolutely evident that there is an increased stress upon the visual system while working on a computer which increases further when it is used as an occupational need. Occupational needs are everything that we do in our life or in other words how we relate to our environment. These occupations include activities that consist of three important properties as follows:

- They actively involve the individual concerned.
- They are meaningful to the individual concerned.
- They include processes that are repetitive in nature.

The straightforward understanding is that visual disturbances caused during a computer task are primarily the effect of work intensity and visual environment of the working station. Setting up a strategy for the assessment of visual performance for computer occupation depends upon the understanding of how visual skills are used in it and the limitations to be appreciated during the process. This comes within the scope of behavioral optometry. Behavioral optometry is an area of understanding which assumes the connection between the visual performance and the occupation.

The work at the office is simply a behavior response to the needs of the environment. Most of the computer-related tasks involve near-vision or extended near-vision tasks. They are repetitive and highly stressful tasks. The computer worker sits in a particular posture for daylong with a mental pressure of targets and occupational performance. The computer games are one step ahead. There is always stress on the sympathetic nervous system for fight-and-flight situation, increasing the secretion of cholesterol and adrenaline and providing no physical relaxation. Many people may not be able to handle the visual stress of prolonged near task and simply cannot deal with computer-related visual stress, resulting in symptoms of CVS.

Visual response is one such behavior. Ninety percent of the interaction with the world is through the vision. In fact, vision leads all our behavioral responses and ironically this is most overlooked. Vision is the function of visual acuity which is a fundamental characteristic of the visual system. In addition to visual acuity, there are many elements of visual system; together, they determine the visual abilities of an individual person. Visual abilities have direct bearing on the visual performance. The extensive use of the visual system while working on computers and its effect in the form of computer vision syndrome have already been established and accepted. The increased complexities of the occupational environments add fuel to this specific demand. Nature has designed our visual system to be so dominant that we adapt our visual system to accommodate any deficiency in the way we see. In the process, we overlook other bodily function abilities and tend to assume typical postures. For a high visually demanding task, the effect is on the entire body. The body adapts to the situation and locates the eyes at a position where they can perform the visual task comfortably resulting in additional stress on bodily muscles. This happens when the typical response does not meet the challenges of the occupation and visual demands exceed the visual abilities; the individual has to modify or adjust his behavior to achieve the required competence. People often forget that the eyes are also one of the many other parts of our body in general. If one of the organs performs well, others will also do so or, in other words, if one aspect of bodily function is healthy, then all others will also be healthy.

Working on a computer for an extensive period of time can lead to visual, ocular, and physical discomfort. The common complaints include eyestrain, headaches, blurred vision, diplopia, sleepiness, difficulty concentrating, loss of comprehension, and pulling sensation. When a patient seeks care for complaints related to computer use, it is important to ensure that enough consideration is being given to visual, visual motor, and visual perceptual skills to address their symptoms. The simple reason is the fact that the problems associated with computer use are very frequent and also affect the total visual system. Most often, they are also associated with physical symptoms.

This implies that a simple refraction and routine ocular examination may not lead us to correct diagnosis and treatment.

Most of the computer-related tasks involve near-vision tasks. Fixation is the primary visual need of any reading task and is followed by depth perception ability. Based upon the above approach, it is possible to devise basic laws as shown in **Flowchart 3.1** on which we can propose an appropriate clinical assessment program for individual reporting with CVS.

- *The computer worker fixates at the target and then follows the same. Fixation and depth perception are, therefore, primary visual skills.*

    This is based on the assumption that fixation is the primary visual ability needed for all reading tasks. Fixation precedes depth perception during reading and depth perception is used to judge how far the text is which is simply controlled by the distance at which it is kept. This distance is determined by the reader. Therefore, very little flexibility is needed in the skill of depth perception. Saccades and regression are two other important visual skills needed for reading tasks.

- *The elements of visual system control the performance of visual skills.*

    The hypothesis is that all the elements of the visual system including visual acuity, contrast sensitivity, accommodative

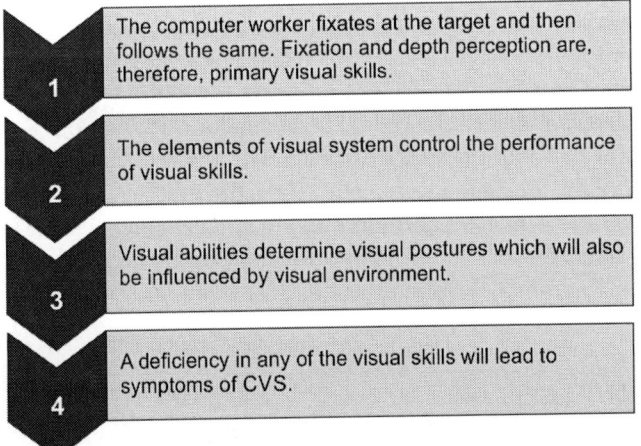

Flowchart 3.1: Laws of computer vision.

1. The computer worker fixates at the target and then follows the same. Fixation and depth perception are, therefore, primary visual skills.
2. The elements of visual system control the performance of visual skills.
3. Visual abilities determine visual postures which will also be influenced by visual environment.
4. A deficiency in any of the visual skills will lead to symptoms of CVS.

system, binocular vision system, oculomotor skills, and color perception ability determine the abilities of the visual system. It follows therefore, if visual deficiency occurs as it may occur because of the visual demands of the close work, it will affect the visual performance and thereby lead to visual symptoms.

- *Visual abilities determine visual postures which will also be influenced by visual environment.*

This is based on the assumption that our visual system is most dominant in receiving information and we alter our bodily posture to accommodate any deficiency in the way our visual system provides us information. For visually intensive tasks, our body locates the eyes at a position where they can perform the visual task comfortably but assumes an awkward posture that results in musculoskeletal problems. Unhygienic visual environment adds to it. The extension of application also includes the constitutional abilities of the computer user as the break point is more readily reached in a feeble than in a robust individual.

- *A deficiency in any of the visual skills will lead to symptoms of CVS.*

The process of vision is a self-directed process. It is driven by conscious decisions and can be explained in the broader framework by **Flowchart 3.2**.

With both eyes open, the process of vision starts when the attention is directed towards an object of the environment and the two eyes move to fixate on the object of interest. Dominant eye leads in fixation which is then followed by nondominant eye. The process is completely driven by eye muscles. The eyes have external and internal muscles. The external muscles fixate the eyes to the point of interest and keep the retinal image in constant motion. Pupil size controls the amount of light that enters the eye and the ciliary muscles control the focusing mechanism. Thus, the precise visual inspection of the object involves accommodation and vergence muscle actions. The oculomotor system maintains fixation using smooth pursuit eye movements, despite object and/or head and body movement.

Flowchart 3.2: Process of vision.

Capturing of object image → Image generation → Fusion of image → Analysis of fused image → Interpretation

The vestibular and muscle proprioceptive system integrates with the visual information to maintain this stability of fixation. If the attention is directed toward another object, a fast, saccadic-jump eye movement is used to establish the new fixation with appropriate accommodation and convergence correction. The cornea and crystalline lens are the refracting elements that make up the imaging components of the visual system. The object in the external environment is imaged on each eye retina. Images are transduced by photoreceptor cells, transforming visible electromagnetic radiation into electrical signals which are transmitted to the visual perception area of brain through the lateral geniculate nucleus. The whole function is under feedback control because the system continually monitors sensory input to check the accuracy of the oculomotor responses in relation to the demands of the task. The visual cortex in the human brain receives these signals where the visual image is processed. The processing within the brain requires the comparison and integration of information received from other sensory organs and a person's past experience.

The motor functions are orchestrated by the brain and, during the visually directed performance, involve eye movement and accommodative-convergence synkinetic coupling adjustments. The task of motor is to bring both foveae onto the object of attention within the visual field and keep them as long as it is required. The motor system also holds the eyes in alignment and clear focus, thereby ensuring the binocular vision. The person can see only one object clearly at any one point. The object seen is clearly the object that the person chooses to make clear. The interpretation placed on visual input is obviously determined by previous experience and learning. The information enables visual processes to operate with minimal attention demand. Maximal attention is then available for interpreting, assimilating, and creatively manipulating the information. Deficiencies in any or all of these basic areas of visual processing can result in overall visual dysfunction.

Based upon the laws of computer vision, a comprehensive clinical evaluation program can be devised as shown in **Flowchart 3.3** for a patient complaining one or more of the symptoms related to CVS.

Usually, it is not necessary to consider a serious underlying etiology when the patient is complaining of one or more symptoms of computer

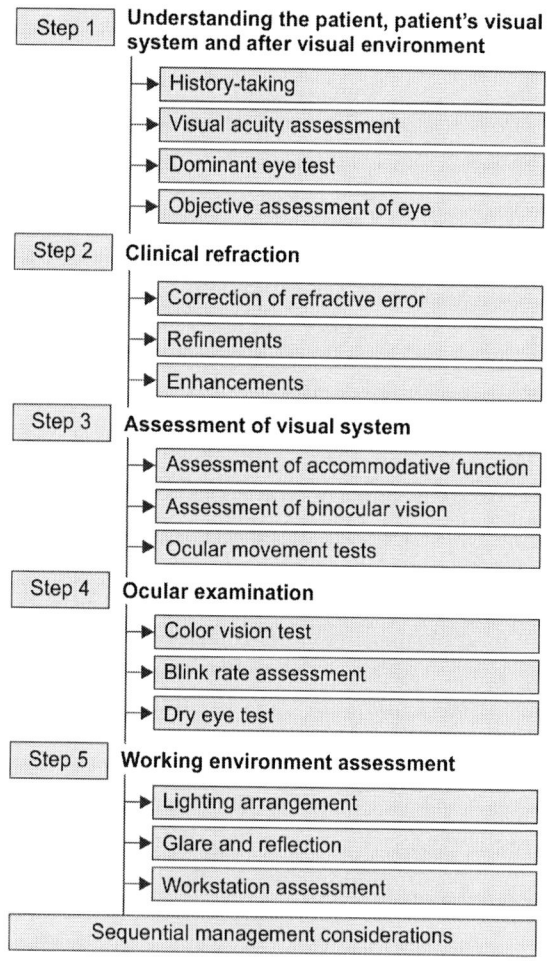

Flowchart 3.3: Clinical evaluation program for a patient reporting symptoms of CVS.

vision syndrome. Visual conditions are associated with a serious underlying disease and usually have an acute onset. They also do not present any health-related history. However, the typical functional disorders that must be ruled out are basic heterophoria, convergence insufficiency, and vergence infacility. Ocular inflammation, such as blepharitis and meibomitis, can cause ocular symptoms of blurred vision after near work. Some of the common clinical signs of patients showing the symptoms of CVS are receded near point of convergence, low amplitude of accommodation, difficulties with plus lenses during binocular and monocular accommodative facility tests, reduced fusional facility, reduced step vergence, etc. However, in practice, most practitioners have been seen to be confined within the realm of uncorrected or undercorrected refractive error and/or dry eyes.

Multiple Choice Questions-Answers

1. Which of the following ocular organs controls the amount of light entering the eye?
   a. Cornea
   b. Pupil
   c. Crystalline lens
   d. Ciliary muscles

2. Which of the following statements is not true?
   a. Dominant eye leads in fixation at the object of interest
   b. The cornea and crystalline lens are the refracting elements of the eye that make up the imaging components of the visual system
   c. The ciliary muscles fixate the eyes to the point of interest and keep the retinal image on constant motion
   d. The photoreceptor cells transform visible electromagnetic radiation into electrical signals which are transmitted to the visual cortex

3. Which of the following is the most common trait of computer-related tasks?
   a. They are near and/or extended near-vision task
   b. They are repetitive and highly visually demanding
   c. They involve the individual concern and are meaningful to them
   d. All of the above

Answer Key

| 1. | (b) | 2. | (c) | 3. | (d) |

Self-Practice Questions

1. Why is it typically not necessary to consider serious underlying etiology in cases of visually related CVS symptoms?
2. Differentiate for a patient the difference between a regular eye examination and a computer vision syndrome evaluation.

CHAPTER 4

Understanding Patient, Patient's Visual Environment, and Visual System

Today, this is an established fact that an effective communication is essential between the patient and the practitioner. The immediate advantage is seen as to improved diagnosis and outcomes, treatment adherence, and patient satisfaction. However, there are challenges from both the sides. Patients come from diverse cultural and ethnic backgrounds and are differently influenced by individual factors related to the psychological and socioeconomic conditions that impact their behavioral responses. On the other hand, the practitioners also try to substitute face-to-face history taking with an intention to minimize time engagement with the patient. This leads to create a strong barrier between them. We need to accept that every patient is unique. He lives in his unique conditions that impact his health. Hence, it is necessary to be familiar with the person and his visual environment before embarking upon the clinical examination procedure. This is especially very important for patients complaining of symptoms of computer vision syndrome (CVS). A patient with symptoms of CVS visits the optometrists; he expects to get the treatment for ocular and/or visual-related difficulties. He may not be very keen in sharing any other symptoms that may not be related directly to vision or visual system, but it may be important for diagnosis. It is, therefore, important to establish a platform where the patient is encouraged to communicate all his symptoms in details and the visual environment in which he works and other related factors. With detailed information about the patient and the status of his vision and visual system, the practitioner can proceed and design an effective treatment plan in which the patient is also involved. The straightforward meaning is that the clinical examination procedure for a patient complaining of symptoms of CVS should start with:

- History taking
- Visual acuity test
- Dominant eye test
- Objective assessment of eyes.

HISTORY TAKING

History taking (**Fig. 4.1**) forms the basic foundation for all medical examination. A well-taken history may lead to make correct diagnosis. The basis of true history taking is good and direct communication between the patient and the practitioner. Sometimes, printed formats are used to expedite the process, but they do not provide the answers to many questions that are obtained through direct observation or interaction with the patient. More importantly, face-to-face contact begins to establish a meaningful patient-practitioner relationship. The patient may begin to relax and feel more confident when he sees that the doctor is taking the time to listen to his complaints. History-taking is an art during which barriers between the patient and the practitioner are broken and a kind of trust is built up and at the end the patient starts taking the practitioner's advice. It is not only important to elicit the critical points of health issues, but it is equally important to demonstrate your expertise. The practitioner also explains the significance of different testing procedures which will follow to elicit his cooperation in forthcoming procedures.

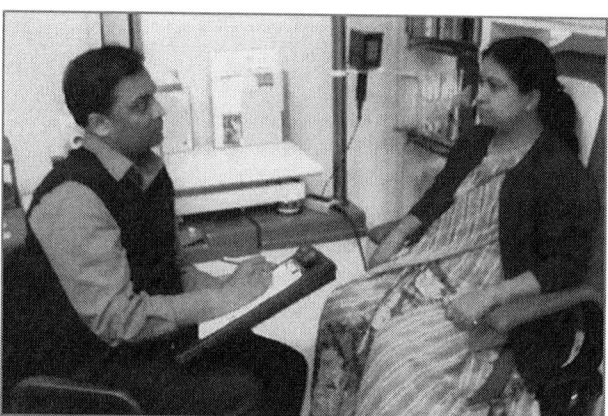

Fig. 4.1: History taking.

History taking also means involving the patient so that he understands his own conditions and better cooperates in the management process. However, the value of the history taking depends upon the ability of the clinician to elicit the relevant information. The sense of what constitutes important information grows with the experience. In most cases, a comprehensive history taking for CVS patients must include what is shown in **Flowchart 4.1**. It requires an ability to listen and apply common sense to define the nature of a particular problem. Extensive history taking is very critical in the successful treatment plan of the patients reporting with the symptoms of CVS. The computer operator needs to understand that visual assessment cannot make things to take a miraculous change, but the potential for improvement is enormous. At the outset, it is usually best to let the patient relate the course of his visual changes and other difficulties and the practitioner should listen without any interruption. This relaxes the patient and he understands that you are interested in the history. Such an understanding at this level sets the tone and encourages support from the patient who relates his own problems to the visual requirements. The proceeding may continue with detailed questioning. The first important issue is to establish the reason for the visit. The practitioner may straightaway ask the patient the reasons for visit and then enquire about his occupations and general lifestyle. With this information, he may proceed to get detailed history about ocular and visual conditions. The following vision-related information is important:

- Do you wear any glasses or contact lenses?
- When was the last eye examination done?
- What was the change in the glass prescription?
- How frequently do your lens power changes?

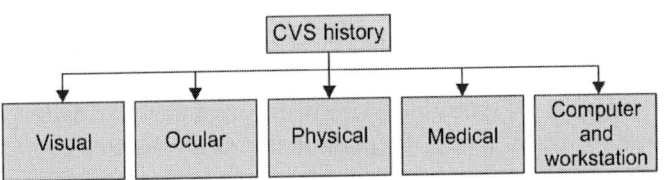

Flowchart 4.1: Comprehensive CVS history taking.

- Do you feel any difficulty in seeing distance after prolonged use of computer?
- Do you see double image?
- Do you frequently lose place when moving eyes between copy and the screen?
- Do you squint while working on computer?
- Do you see any changes in color perception?

In addition, you may ask questions that are related to dry eyes, for example, presence of dryness in eyes, irritated eyes, and foreign-body sensation. History of past eye treatment or surgery is also important. With this information, the practitioner may set to ask questions related to general health such as neck pain, shoulder pain, back pain, muscles ache, wrist and finger stiffness, and headache during or after computer work that will straightaway direct toward the diagnosis. In addition, information about hypertension and diabetes and intake of antidepressant drugs are important to note. The history is so taken enough to direct you to diagnosis, and hence you may complete the process of history taking with the following set of questions:

- Placement of computer monitor
- Working distance and viewing angle
- Types of chair—with footrest, without footrest, handle, and back support
- Types of room—lighting and their arrangement
- Room paint types—matt, glossy, plain, or with stripes
- Location of window
- Tabletop—glass, wooden, matt, or shining
- Approximate duration of time spent on computer
- Types of monitor used
- Size and form of screen characters
- Screen color
- Contrast and brightness of monitor

All information so elicited must be recorded on a standardized form and should be used to relate to clinical signs. It is also advised not to spend too long time taking history as it may lead to the patient getting frustrated and the patient stands unsatisfied right at the beginning.

VISUAL ACUITY TEST

Visual acuity is the fundamental characteristic of the visual system and is the prime determinant of any regime that aims to improve visual and therefore occupational performance. It is the time-dependent measurement of retinal health and is specified by date and time on which assessment took place. Visual acuity needs to be recorded in three states of condition as shown in **Flowchart 4.2**.

High- and Low-Contrast Acuity

High- and low-contrast acuity measurements are important measurements to understand the insights of the visual system. High-contrast acuity measurement becomes a benchmark against which the benefits of using refractive correction may be referred. Low-contrast acuity is more likely to elicit a visual deficiency. Low-contrast acuity test is the useful tool in the early detection of various diseases as well as in the determination of any complications. Two persons with similar acuity can function differently that may be predicted by differentiating between high- and low-contrast acuity. In general, a poor performance with low-contrast acuity points toward the need for more attention to glare control, contrast of viewing targets, and the illumination.

Visual Acuity with Current Correction

A well-taken visual acuity measurement is critical to ensuring an accurate spectacle correction—just right ... not too strong ... and not too weak. This implies that the examiner is looking for the finest detail that the visual system can resolve. Measuring the visual acuity with the existing correction reveals information as to the possibilities of any improvements. Many times, the patient carries a perception that his

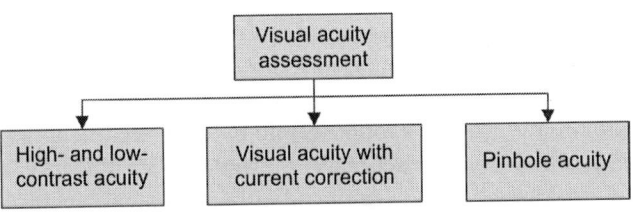

Flowchart 4.2: Visual acuity tests.

acuity is better with his old correction than the new one. Recording the acuity with old correction provides an opportunity to compare with the new correction and is also a strong indicator on which the subjective refraction may be initiated.

Pinhole Acuity

Pinhole acuity is critical to determine whether the decreased visual acuity is correctable by lenses or not. It reduces the size of the blur circle that has been created on the retina by an uncorrected refractive error that establishes that better visual acuity may be achieved with refraction. However, for most CVS patients, this may not be very important, but it is certainly helpful for differential diagnosis.

DOMINANT EYE TEST

Something happens—that is one thing. Why it happens and what it amounts to, these are entirely different things. People easily misinterpret knowingly or unknowingly just because the implication of a concept is not clear and well established.

The phenomenon of "dominant eye" probably falls in this category. The concept has been known for several years, but its implications are still not very clear. We all know that most people are born with a dominant tendency to use one eye more than the other even if the vision in both eyes is perfect. In the binocular vision system, one eye leads in fixating at the target and the other follows the leading eye. There is a small time lag between the two eyes fixating at the same target that allows the required depth perception. The phenomenon suggests that the leading eye is sighting first toward the target and, therefore, it may be considered as sighting dominant eye, the other being the nondominant eye. Thus, eye dominancy refers to the superiority of one eye over the other in terms of receiving the visual inputs. It contributes most to the visual perception. It is easier in general to suppress the nondominant eye. For example, while lining up two objects one relies on the dominant eye even if the nondominant eye is also open. Some patients are uncomfortable if their dominant eye is fractionally blurred or over plus by 0.25 Dsph relative to the other eye. On the other hand, a small uncorrected or residual refractive error in the nondominant eye may possibly not give any discomfort. Law 1 of "laws of computer vision" says that fixation is the primary visual ability for the person working on a computer. If the fixating eye is not adequately corrected, it may lose its place and may wander leading to loss of place. Knowing the sighted dominant eye is, therefore, critical to the tasks where visual demands are at peak. Establishing which eye is dominant plays a vital role in binocular vision assessment. It may help us to design a better visual behavioral pattern. For example, for people working more on computer, the location of the visual target plays a major role in determining sitting posture. Visual requirements result in the user positioning the body so that the face is parallel to the viewing surface. This principle should be remembered when determining placement of the monitor and allied attachments. Document holders are generally placed to the side of or in front of the monitor. When placing the document holder to the side of the monitor, the dominant eye should be considered. Favoring the dominant eye with the most frequently used visual targets may require less eye, head, neck, and body movement to view these targets. This is due to the fact that the center of the visual field is closer to the dominant eye than the nondominant eye. A left-eye-dominant person should position frequently viewed documents to the left of the monitor.

The majority of the population is right-eye-dominant; some are left-eye-dominant also. A small number of people also show no definite ocular dominancy. Eye dominance is believed to be congenital, showing a consistent preference from the early infancy. Although both eyes are used to judge the distance, it is the alignment of the usually dominant eye and the target that gives the direction. It implies that eye dominancy is an important phenomenon for highly visually demanding tasks.

There are various methods to assess eye dominance. The "hole in the card test" **(Fig. 4.2)** is the simplest among them. The subject is given a card with a small hole of 25 mm in the middle and is instructed to hold it with both hands stretched out. He is then instructed to view a distant object through the hole with both eyes open. If binocular vision is present, he tends to center the hole between his eyes. The observer then observes his eyes through the hole by alternately closing his eyes. The eye is seen through the hole which would be the dominant eye of the person.

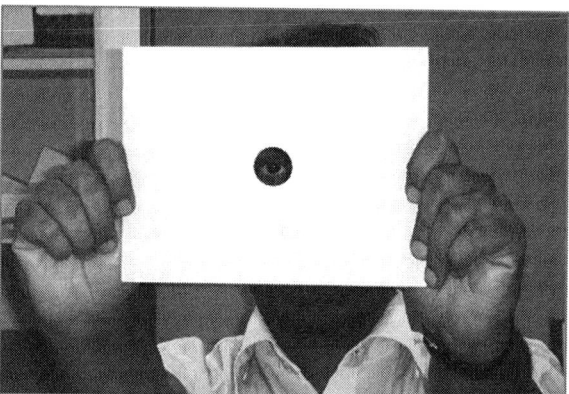

Fig. 4.2: Hole in the card test.

Alternatively, the observer may ask the patient to slowly draw the opening back to the head to determine which eye is viewing the object. Invariably, the patient will take the hole toward his dominant eye.

OBJECTIVE ASSESSMENT OF EYE

Objective assessment of eye gives a good starting point to the practitioner on which the practitioner can set the platform for the comprehensive eye examination. The practitioner performs the gross observation of the anterior structures of the eyes and determines the refractive error without taking any input from the patient and thus establishes a baseline idea to carry out the subjective refraction. Several tests form the part of the objective assessment of the eyes. The common tests that may be applied for patients complaining of symptoms related to CVS are shown in **Flowchart 4.3**.

Torchlight Examination

Torchlight is a wonderful tool to carry out the gross examination of the anterior segment of the eye. It is a very effective tool to detect distinct abnormalities and can be very effective in differential diagnosis. Pen light is commonly used for the purpose.

A direct focusing of pen light or asking the patient to fixate at the pen light helps detecting strabismus by the Hirschberg corneal light reflex. You just need to examine the exact location of the bright light

Flowchart 4.3: Tests for objective assessment of eye.

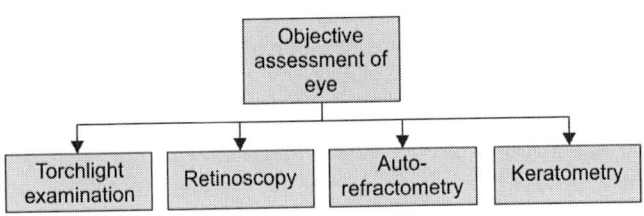

reflex on the cornea near the center of the pupil and compare both eyes. In normal eyes, when the eyes are looking straight ahead, the Hirschberg reflex will be seen at the same position of both eyes, i.e., 5° toward nasally. Esotrope will show reflex toward the ear away from nose.

Pupil shape, size, and reactivity to light can be examined with pen light. Under normal illumination, the normal pupil size is 3–4 mm. Both eyes' pupils are of the same shape and size. Pupillary light reflex test also provides useful information about the integrity of the sensory and motor functions of the eye. Under normal condition, pupils of both eyes respond identically to a light stimulus, regardless of which eye is being stimulated. Both pupils should constrict with light shone onto either eye alone. If light is being shone on the right pupil, the response seen in the right eye is direct response and the response seen in the left eye is consensual response. Direct response in the right eye without a consensual response in the left eye implies a problem with the motor connection to the left eye. Lack of direct response implies a problem with sensory inputs from the right eye.

A gross idea of anterior chamber depth can be made with the help of pen light. The flashlight is shone from the temporal side onto the cornea, parallel but anterior to the iris. A shadow on the nasal limbus identifies the eye with a shallow anterior chamber, i.e., at the risk of closure. It is also important to remember that this is not the conclusive confirmation of angle closure, but should be referred for gonioscopy for further evaluation.

A gross examination of iris color can also be done with pen light. A difference in color between the two irises may be indicative of congenital abnormalities. Normal sclera is white and opaque and fibrous structure. Blue discoloration may be because of scleral thinning and underlying prominence of dark choroid.

Retinoscopy

Since the introduction of retinoscopy, it has been performed as one of the very first procedures during the eye examination. It is a great tool to establish a strong basis for the refractive status of the eye on which subjective refraction can be followed. In addition, retinoscopy helps to detect the aberrations of the cornea and the crystalline lens. It also provides some clues in respect of opacities of ocular media. Retinoscopy is particularly a very helpful tool with uncooperative or malingering patients, infants, deaf, and in all those cases where language or communication creates difficulties during the process of refraction.

Autorefractometry

Autorefractometer is an automated, fast, and very reliable method of objective refraction. The results obtained from the autorefractometer are highly repeatable. It not only provides several estimates of the refractive error but also suggests an average reading that can be used as a basis for subjective evaluation of the refractive error. The procedure takes hardly a few seconds. Several readings are taken which the machine averages to form a prescription. No feedback is required from the patient during this process. Within few seconds, an approximate measurement of a person's prescription can be made by the machine and printed out.

Keratometry

Keratometry is an instrument used to measure the front surface curvature of the cornea. The readings provide information as to the corneal astigmatism which may be used as baseline cylinder correction needed for the patient. However, the amount of astigmatism derived by a keratometer may differ from that of spectacle refraction. It may be more than the spectacle refraction or less than the spectacle refraction or may be same. Besides, it can also provide qualitative assessment of tear film and corneal integrity.

Chapter 4: Understanding Patient, Patient's Visual Environment... 41

Multiple Choice Questions-Answers

1. When recording a patient's history who is complaining of symptoms of CVS, which of the following information is not relevant?
   a. Details regarding difficulties in light/dark adaptation
   b. Any difficulties in bright light
   c. Details regarding office-lighting arrangement and workstation ergonomics
   d. Whether there is any history of ARMD

2. Which of the following statements is true regarding keratometry?
   a. It measures the curvature of the anterior surface of cornea
   b. It provides information as to the proportion of corneal astigmatism
   c. It provides the qualitative assessment of tear film and corneal integrity
   d. All of the above

3. Which of the following statements is not true?
   a. Pupil should constrict with light shone onto either eyes alone
   b. Lack of direct pupil response to light shone implies a problem with sensory inputs from the eye and lack of indirect pupil response to light implies problem with motor connection to fellow eye
   c. Normal Hirschberg reflex is seen at 5° toward the temporal side at the same position of both eyes
   d. A difference in color between the irises of the two eyes may indicate congenital abnormalities

4. Which of the following is correct about retinoscopy?
   a. It gives the initial view of the inside of the eye
   b. It helps to know the refractive status of the eye
   c. It is not dependent upon the subject's response
   d. All of the above

Answer Key

| 1. | (d) | 2. | (d) | 3. | (c) | 4. | (d) |

Self-Practice Questions

1. Why is it important to know the patient and patient's visual environment before deciding the treatment plan for cases of CVS?
2. How do visual demands for people working with visual display units use differ from those of sports athletes and players? Also, explain taking clues from common lifestyle of general population.

CHAPTER 5

Correction of Refractive Error for Computer Vision Syndrome Patient

SYMPTOMS

A patient with uncorrected or undercorrected refractive error most commonly shows the following symptoms:
- He blinks excessively during the near task.
- He frowns, scowls, or squints to see distance target.
- He avoids reading work.
- He fatigues easily during visual task.
- He rubs his eyes during or after visual activity.
- He complains of blur vision while reading or writing.

RATIONALE

The first consideration for all patients with vision-related complaints is to correct refractive error. An uncorrected refractive error will lead to deficiency in visual skills and according to Law 4 of "Laws of Computer Vision," any deficiency in visual skills will lead to symptoms of CVS. This, in turn, will affect occupational performance. The straightforward meaning is that uncorrected refractive error of any magnitude is very critical for people working on a computer. The reasons are simple. Computer tasks are highly visually demanding tasks requiring focused concentration with reduced blink rate and widening of the eyelids. The condition is exacerbated by low humidity and drying atmosphere of the working station. The cumulative effect is on the visual function of the computer workers because of its effect on various elements of the visual system:
- It influences the accommodative function of the eyes.
- It influences the vergence function of the eyes.

- It creates an imbalance between the two eyes, leading to sensory fusion disturbances.

Sometimes, even a small degree of refractive error may prove to be significant to cause symptoms because of the following possibilities:
- The patient reports significant accommodative and binocular vision problem. In such a case, correcting the low refractive error becomes very important as it will improve fusion and assist in the management.
- Another possibility is that the patient has low refractive error, and all his accommodative and binocular vision evaluation are within expected values. In such a case, the clinician has no other choice than to prescribe for the low refractive error.

Experience shows that there is often an accommodative, ocular motor, or binocular vision disorder present in addition to low refractive error. It is very unusual to find a low refractive error in isolation that accounts for significant symptoms.

TYPES OF REFRACTIVE ERROR

The common refractive error includes hypermetropia, myopia, and astigmatism.

Hypermetropia

Hypermetropia is farsightedness. The patient can accommodate and can correct his error. A young individual who has large accommodative amplitude can correct even a large amount of hypermetropia. But he cannot manage to see at near as the entire accommodative ability is spent while distance viewing. However, the amplitude of accommodation decreases with age and compensating for hypermetropic error with accommodation becomes difficult even for distance. The straightforward understanding is that uncorrected hypermetropia is a very important cause of eyestrain. Latent hypermetropia can be uncovered with cycloplegic refraction, in which one's accommodative power is eliminated with eye drops. Without cycloplegic refraction, he may be mistakably prescribed bifocals when the reading problem is reported. Proper hypermetropic correction in these cases will make the patient more comfortable at all times and also may postpone the need for bifocal glasses.

Myopia

Myopes are shortsighted. They can see at near working distance even without correction. Thus, myopia, by itself, does not usually cause symptoms for a computer user. Low-to-moderate myopic individuals can read comfortably without their correction at normal viewing distance. A myope with –2.50D can read at 40 cm without using his accommodation. However, he may experience difficulties while viewing at the computer monitor because a computer monitor is located farther away than normal reading distance. In order to compensate for the same, they may assume an awkward posture to obtain a shorter distance to the computer screen and thus may show the symptoms of CVS.

Astigmatism

Astigmatism creates blur vision at all working distances. A small amount of astigmatism may not be noticed in normal life. But when the visual demand increases as occurs while working on computers, playing sports at higher levels, etc., it may affect visual performance. Sometimes, the individual may feel headache or eyestrain. Studies have shown that an uncorrected astigmatic error of 0.50D is significantly associated with visual discomfort for work at computer displays. Therefore, astigmatism of 0.50D or greater should always be considered as a potential problem for a computer user and should be corrected.

CYCLOPLEGIC REFRACTION

A cycloplegic refraction is the procedure used to determine a patient's true refractive error by temporarily paralyzing the muscles that aid in focusing using cycloplegic drops. Dry subjective refraction is sufficient to determine the refractive error in most cases. But when esophoria is present or latent hypermetropia is suspected, a cycloplegic refraction may be more helpful. Esodeviation tends to be associated with a greater amount of hypermetropia. By prescribing the maximum plus, we can attempt to minimize a possible underlying etiologic factor. The following care must be taken while performing cycloplegic refraction:
- Cycloplegic refraction should be conducted after completing all other eye tests.

- The patient's only distance vision correction is being done after cycloplegia. Near vision is not examined as accommodation is being suspended. Near vision must be checked during manifest refraction prior to cycloplegia.
- When performing cycloplegic refraction, it is possible that occasionally the patient may not refract to the same visual acuity that has been arrived at during the manifest refraction. This may be because the dilated eye lacks the pinhole effect of small pupil.

REFRACTIVE ERROR CORRECTION

Good refraction is in fact the primary requirement in achieving the optimal visual performance. Unless visual acuity is maximized during the refraction, all other aspects of clinical care have no meaning and this is more critical when there is a pressure of excess visual demands on the visual system. The theoretical aim of the refraction is to prescribe a pair of lenses that ensure the retina to be in conjugate with optical infinity. But the true objective of the refraction is to provide the patient with a correction that provides him clear and comfortable vision and to which he adapts quickly and allows him to work for a longer period of time without any symptoms. Therefore, the mechanics of refraction should not only aim to enhance the vision but also focus to minimize the disadvantage to establish a sustained comfortable visual performance. There are three important stages that are critical for a patient with symptoms of CVS as shown in **Flowchart 5.1**.

Subjective Refraction

Now with comprehensive information about the present condition of the visual system and results of objective refraction in hand, the

Flowchart 5.1: Correction of refractive error, sequential steps.

```
                    Refractive
                 error correction
          ┌──────────────┼──────────────┐
     Subjective       Refinements    Enhancements
     refraction
```

Chapter 5: Correction of Refractive Error for Computer... 47

practitioner gathers all the information about the patient's history, his chief complaints, and current status of the visual system and relate all collected information, make a judgment as to the further course of action, and decide a goal for the treatment. A quick and in-depth brain-storming exercise is needed to relate the symptoms to the objective assessment results before embarking upon the monocular subjective refraction. Subjective refraction is a method of estimating the refractive error wherein the patient's response is important before arriving at the results. The ultimate goal is to arrive at a combination of lenses that result in maximum visual acuity. The following points form the important elements of the process:

- Subjective refraction is initiated by selecting an initial trial lens which may be based on the following factors:
  o Current lens prescription of the patient
  o A set of lenses you decide based on your initial data collection
  o It may be the results of autorefractometer or retinoscope.
- Once the initial trial lens is put in the trial frame, you ask the patient to look at the Distance Vision Test Chart through a lens power one step stronger or one step weaker and ask which one appears clearer to him. Depending upon the lens the patient chooses, you compare another combination of one step stronger or one step weaker.
- In case spherical and cylinder both are there in the trial frame, it is prudent to check the axis first and then the amount of cylinder correction and finally the spherical correction needed.
- In case of high astigmatic correction, a stenopaic slit is a very effective tool to decide the axis of cylinder and amount of cylinder.
- Measure the vertex distance in high refractive error above −5.00D for myopes and above +4.00D for hyperopes as the effect of prescribed minus power will reduce if the vertex distance increases and it will increase with plus lens. When you measure the vertex distance, do not forget to mention the same in the prescription.
- Avoid large changes in prescription; do not change spherical by more than 0.75D, cylinder by more than 0.50D, and axis by more than 10°. Excess changes call for counseling for probable problems. Whenever you get a major change in the cylinder or the axis, do not forget to check for aniseikonic effect.

- If the distance visual acuity in two eyes is significantly different, determine the near addition for each eye separately and reverify it binocularly.
- Do not forget to ask the patient's habitual near working distance while checking the near addition. Be careful while prescribing near addition to a patient below the age of 38–40 years just because it makes the text clearer. Rule out the possibility of latent hypermetropia or esophoria.
- The most common mistake that an examiner makes while doing refraction is giving the person more minus. This is because adding a small amount of extra minus power may not make the vision worse if the person can accommodate. He may say that his vision looks the same or sometimes better. In such cases, the patient may complain of asthenopia after wearing them for longer hours of time. Sometimes, symptoms may be so bad that the person will not be able to wear the spectacles.
- Fogging method is very effective in case of hypermetropia, especially if it is for the first time. One can also look for cycloplegic refraction in such cases.

Refinements

The final results of the subjective refraction are arrived at and the results of the completed tests are to be refined. Two clinical tests are usually performed for the purpose—one aims to refine the results monocularly and the other aims to ensure that the results of monocular subjective refraction work binocularly without any problem. The two tests are:
1. Duochrome test for spherical endpoint
2. Binocular balancing.

The examiner needs to keep in mind that over-minus will stimulate accommodation and over-plus will blur the vision. Duochrome test for spherical endpoint is performed to refine the spherical correction or to determine the spherical endpoint of the refractive error after the subjective refraction is completed. The test has to be done under complete darkness as it reduces veiling luminance and dilates the pupil, thereby increasing the chromatic aberration and making the test more effective. It is important to control the accommodation by slight fogging. Add +0.25Dsph lens monocularly before asking the patient to notice the difference between letters of two backgrounds. The test is very sensitive to even a small change of 0.25D. The plus sphere is reduced until letters on both the backgrounds appear equally distinct. The next reduction of only 0.25D makes letters on the green background more distinct. Ideally, the spherical endpoint should be decided when the letters on the red background are comparatively sharper.

Binocular balancing is performed to equalize the stimulus to accommodation for the two eyes. The two most common procedures which are normally used are:
1. Alternate occlusion test
2. Prism dissociated test.

The test has to be done under standard room lights. If balancing is not possible, leave the patient at a point which produces least difference. The dominant eye is left with little clearer vision.

Enhancements

Good visual acuity is the first essential criterion for symptom-free performance and visual comfort while working on a computer display. In many cases, simply an accurate correction of refractive error for working on a computer monitor may relieve the symptoms. Therefore, it is a prudent idea to think differently for correcting refractive error for people working on computers. The following ideas may provide better results:
- Traditionally, refraction is done at a distance of 20 feet for distance vision and for near at a distance of 40 cm. One of the most important factors for computer users is the allowance for the distance at which the monitor is placed. Typically, we are dealing with subjects who need good acuity at a distance which is neither a standard long distance nor a standard near-vision distance. Leaving them with correction at 6 meters and 40 cm may not give them sufficient flexibility. Probably, it may be prudent to check the refractive correction at several distances: from the eyes to the middle of the screen or even lower onto the keyboard or to the source document, depending upon the respective use of the distance more often. The most challenging refraction problem is

with presbyopic patients. They suffer discomfort from having to shift their gaze between different parts of the multifocal lenses or between pair of spectacles. Consideration should be given to prescribe them a separate prescription for computer distance either in the form of bifocal glasses or any other occupational lenses. This is discussed in more detail in another chapter. In addition, it is also helpful to know how frequently the user looks away from the screen or other work surfaces.

- The electronically generated letter types that are displayed on computer screens are made of pixels. These pixelated letters have poorly defined edges. They are brightest in the center and diminish in contrast at the edges. Human eyes and brain react very well to the most printed materials that have good contrast, whereas they react differently to those pixelated characters. They are optically imperfect characters, and sometimes even the perfectly functioning eyes have difficulties maintaining accurate focus on such imperfect characters. They may alter the results of the refraction correction for such a highly visually demanding task.
- The pixelated nature of the letters may also add demand on the accommodative mechanism. The increased demand on accommodative mechanism often interacts with the refractive error. It is, therefore, very important not to avoid even the smallest amount of the refractive correction.
- A computer worker uses his accommodation mechanism and convergence ability constantly while working on computers. During the process, pupil constriction also occurs. Small pupil reduces the total effect of higher order aberration and increases the depth of focus. The patient is usually not in such a posture during refraction with the Snellen test type held at 20 feet.

There seems to be an effect of many factors on the refractive error of the computer users. Unfortunately, not much of the studies are available. However, we cannot overlook that the primary reason for correcting refractive error is to obtain an improvement in visual acuity so that the patient can see clearly and comfortably. More studies will definitely change the scenario of refractive error correction for computer users.

Chapter 5: Correction of Refractive Error for Computer...

Multiple Choice Questions-Answers

1. Which of the following may be less than optimal in the presence of significant uncorrected refractive error?
   a. Fixation skill
   b. Saccades
   c. Pursuits
   d. All of the above

2. Which of the following statements is not true for cycloplegic refraction?
   a. Cycloplegic refraction is usually conducted after completing all other eye tests
   b. Cycloplegic refraction indicates the magnitude of refractive error and noncycloplegic refraction indicates the acceptability
   c. Only distance correction is being done under cycloplegia and near-vision is not examined
   d. Same visual acuity is always achieved with cycloplegic refraction as achieved during manifest subjective refraction

3. If a refractive error is not fully corrected, it may lead to:
   a. Either under- or overaccommodation
   b. Unusual demand of either negative or positive fusional vergence
   c. Decreased fusional ability as a result of blurred retinal images
   d. All of the above

Answer Key

| 1. | (d) | 2. | (d) | 3. | (d) |

Self-Practice Questions

1. Explain why correcting refracting error is an important first step when treating a computer-related vision problem.
2. How can different types of visual skills be affected in the presence of significantly uncorrected refractive error? Explain in light of symptoms of CVS.

CHAPTER 6

Accommodative Function and its Management

SYMPTOMS

A patient with disorder in accommodation function shows the following symptoms in common:
- He complains blurring at distance after persistent near work.
- He complains of intermittent near blurring.
- Asthenopia
- Headache

RATIONALE

Prolonged viewing of a computer display puts huge demand on the accommodative mechanism which often interacts with refractive error. The uninterrupted constant gaze at the computer display locks the accommodative mechanism at the near-viewing distance that delays the accommodation-relaxing ability of the eyes when they look at a distance after an extended work on the computer display. The ciliary muscle remains locked in the near-contracted position. This effectively makes the eyes myopic when looking at distance. As the ciliary muscles start functioning properly, distance objects become clear in a few seconds. Thus, post-near work, there is a delay in focusing at distance. Intermittent near-blurring is normally because of ill-sustained accommodation at computer viewing distance. The eyes find it difficult to maintain steady focus on the near targets. The symptoms aggravate as the day passes. While working on a computer display, the excess demand on the accommodation mechanism puts extra stress on ciliary muscles. The ciliary muscles have to work much harder to focus on the monitor. The constant flexing of ciliary muscles

Chapter 6: Accommodative Function and its Management

creates fatigue and generates tired eyes. In addition, accommodation is also associated with convergence which puts extra demand on extraocular muscles. The condition can affect visual comfort, and the patient may show the symptoms of asthenopia and headache. The overall impact is on the total accommodation system, and according to Law 2 of the "Laws of Computer Vision" the elements of the visual system control the performance of visual skills. Accommodative ability is adversely affected that deteriorates the performance of visual skills. The constant focusing on computer display and allied near work puts extra pressure on the accommodative function, leading to visual deficiency. Law 4 of the "Laws of Computer Vision" says that a deficiency in any of the visual skills will lead to symptoms of CVS.

ACCOMMODATIVE FUNCTION

Accommodation determines the focusing ability of the eyes. The process allows the eyes to change its optical power so that it can maintain a clear image or focus on an object as its distance varies. **Figures 6.1A and B** show the two states of the eye. **Figure 6.1A** shows the condition when the eye is relaxed and **Figure 6.1B** shows the condition when the eye is accommodated. When a person views a far object, the ciliary muscles relax allowing the lens zonules and suspensory ligaments to create a pull on the lens to flatten it. The eye power is reduced and is able to focus onto the object of regard at distance. When the viewing gaze shifts to a near object, the ciliary

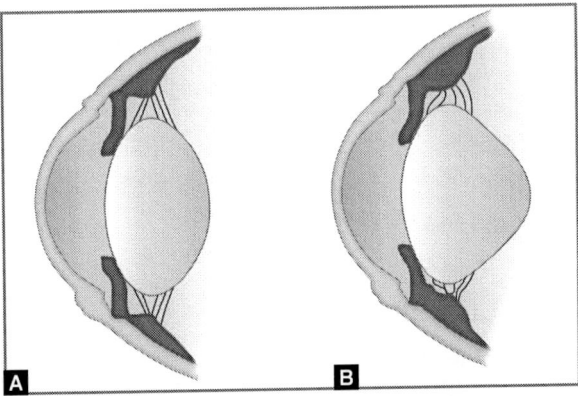

Figs. 6.1A and B: Two states of eye: (A) Relaxed eye; (B) Accommodated eye.

muscles contract causing the lens zonules to relax that allow the lens to take a thicker and more convex form so that it can focus on near object. Thus, accommodation provides the retina with a clear, sharp image of the objects at various distances. Accommodation acts as a stimulus that also produces a change in the relative position of the visual axis as a response, the angle formed by the visual axis increases, and the eyes converge. In addition, with fixation shifted at near distance, miosis occurs, resulting in pupil constriction.

Accommodation is measured in diopters (D), which is the reciprocal of the fixation distance. The young human eye can change focus from infinity to as near as 6.5 cm from the eyes, which is the reciprocal of fixation distance in meters and corresponds in diopter.

$$\text{Accommodation} = \frac{1}{\text{Fixation distance in meters}} D$$

Table 6.1 shows the amount of accommodation exerted at various distances.

The mechanism of accommodation develops by 4 months of age. Accommodative ability decreases with age, being maximum at a very young age and gradually decreasing as we grow in age. Around the middle age, the reduction of the accommodative ability reaches to a level to such an extent that the individual is unable to focus on the near object, leading to the onset of presbyopia.

Accommodation is remarkably a quick response to a stimulus. When the retina receives a stimulus to accommodate, the reaction time of the response initiated is quite short. The reaction time for

Table 6.1: Amount of accommodation at different fixation distances.

Fixation distance	Amount of accommodation
6 meters	0.17D
5 meters	0.20D
4 meters	0.25D
3 meters	0.33D
2 meters	0.50D
1 meter	1.00D

"far to near" accommodation has been recorded to be approximately 0.29 seconds to a response time of about 0.75 seconds to reach the steady state. The same for "near to far" has been approximated to be in the range of 0.35–1.19 seconds. When the target is moved slowly so that the process of defocusing is gradual, the accommodation does not change continuously but in oscillatory fluctuations so that the extent of the accommodation is not always correct.

Accommodation is not a static condition. Microfluctuations constantly occur in the degree of accommodation of the nonpresbyopic eye. The magnitude of these fluctuations is very small. These microfluctuations occur during accommodation and also to a minute degree when the accommodation is relaxed. The fluctuations in accommodation seem obviously due to the normal activity of the ciliary muscle and are comparable to the motor tremor seen in all muscles. This is seen in the eye in the constant variations in the diameter of the pupil and the movement of the globe which prevent absolute fixation.

Accommodative response is usually more accurate when viewing higher spatial frequencies than when viewing lower ones. Studies have suggested that the pixelated nature of characters from the video display may negatively affect the accommodative response creating extra strain on the accommodative mechanism that results in a decrease in amplitude of accommodation (AA) and accommodative fluctuations at the end of the day. When an individual works for longer hours at a stretch on the computer display, the muscles actually spasm so that the crystalline lens stay overfocused. This creates a temporary myopia, creating difficulties to refocus at a distance object. Thus, accommodative anomalies occur that include the conditions as shown in **Flowchart 6.1**.

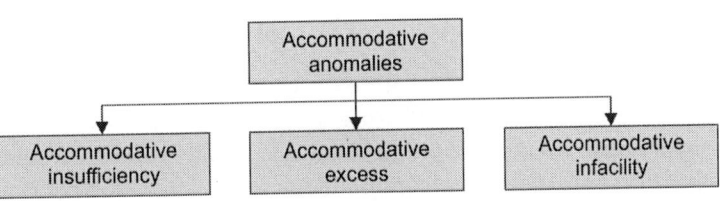

Flowchart 6.1: Accommodative anomalies.

Accommodative Insufficiency

The condition is characterized by reduced amplitude of accommodation than the lower limit of the expected value for the patient's age. The patient finds it difficult to stimulate accommodation, not to be confused with presbyopia, where AA is not abnormal relative to age; rather, it is low to permit clear, comfortable near-vision. Ill-sustained accommodations where the amplitude of accommodation is normal under a typical test, but reduces over time, and accommodative paralysis or paresis are associated conditions. Ill-sustained accommodation also causes intermittent blur at computer viewing distance.

Accommodative Excess

The condition occurs when the accommodative response exceeds the accommodative stimulus. The patient has difficulty with all tasks requiring relaxation of accommodation. The symptom aggravates as the day passes. When an individual works for longer hours at a stretch on the computer display, the muscles actually spasm so that the crystalline lens stay overfocused. This creates a temporary myopia, creating difficulties to refocus at a distance object. Hence, a computer user complains of a temporary blur at a distance after prolonged near work.

Accommodative Infacility

Accommodative infacility is the inability of the patient to rapidly change the accommodative response from one level to another. Accommodative dynamics are slowed. The patient experiences difficulty changing the accommodative responses. It occurs only with effort and difficulties. The computer user finds it difficult to look at the source document located at one point to the computer display located at the other point quickly and easily. Amplitude of accommodation is normal, but the patient's ability to make use of this amplitude quickly and for a longer period of time is inadequate.

CLINICAL EXAMINATION OF ACCOMMODATION FUNCTION

An eye examination of a computer worker for the assessment of accommodative function must be performed before instilling mydriatic or cycloplegic pharmaceuticals, and it includes the tests of the different aspects of accommodation as shown in **Flowchart 6.2:**

Flowchart 6.2: Elements of accommodation function.

```
                    Clinical tests for
                 accommodation function
        ┌───────────────┬──────────────┬───────────────┐
  Amplitude of    Accommodative    Binocular        Lag of
  accommodation      facility    Accommodative   accommodation
                                    range
```

Amplitude of Accommodation

Amplitude of accommodation (AA) measures the ability of an individual, to focus clearly on the object at a near distance. Monocular expected amplitude of accommodation is the function of age and is given by the Hofstetter formula:

AA = 15–0.25 (x)

Where x = patient's age in years.

Table 6.2 shows the average amplitude of accommodation, in diopter, for a given age as estimated by the Hofstetter formula.

If the measured amplitude is reduced because of the patient's age to a level below 5.00D, and the patient has difficulty reading, then the patient is said to have presbyopia. Age-related decline in accommodation occurs universally and by 60 years of age, most of the population will have noticed a decrease in their ability to focus on close objects.

Amplitude of accommodation also varies with the gaze angle of the eye, generally being greatest with the eye gazing down and least with upward gaze.

Table 6.2: Amplitude of accommodation as the age varies.

Age	Amplitude of accommodation
10 years	12.50D
20 years	10.00D
30 years	7.50D
40 years	5.00D
50 years	2.50D
60 years	0.00D

The tests to measure amplitude of accommodation are usually performed with each eye separately. A target with a small detail is slowly moved toward the eye and the patient is instructed to note first detectable blur point which is measured from the spectacle plane in meters and then converted into diopter. The most common tests are:
- Push-up amplitude
- Minus lens test

Patients with poor amplitude of accommodation than expected values show accommodative insufficiency and usually demonstrate poor accommodative sustaining ability.

Accommodative Facility

Accommodative facility is the ability of the patient to rapidly change the accommodative response from one level to another **(Fig. 6.2)**. It is the measure of ease and quickness with which the accommodation of the eye can change from one accommodative state to another. This is a very good indicator of accommodative function and should be run on all pre-presbyopic patients with symptoms. The test to measure accommodative facility evaluates the stamina and dynamics of accommodative response. The tests should be performed monocularly as well as binocularly. Binocular testing is an assessment of the interactions between accommodation and vergence and is not the pure measurement of accommodative facility. If the patient experiences difficulties with binocular testing, then monocular testing

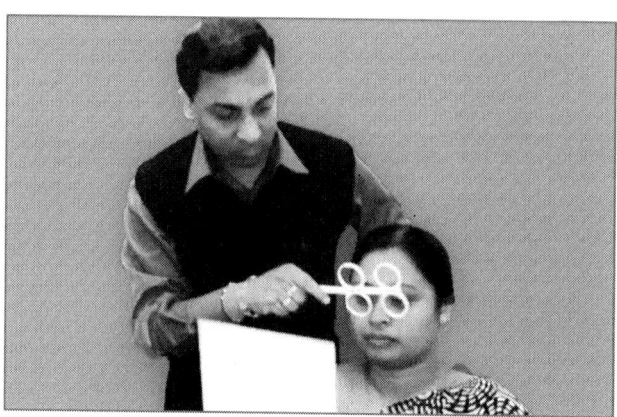

Fig. 6.2: Testing of the accommodative facility.

may also be administered, which would be diagnostic in such case. The patient views a target with small detail. The following tests are administered using the lens flippers of + and −1.50D or + and −2.00D before the eyes:
- Binocular accommodative facility (BAF)
- Monocular accommodative facility (MAF)

The expected performance for 1.50D flipper is 10 cpm with both eyes and 13 cpm monocularly. For + and −2.00D flipper, it is 11 cpm with both eyes and 8 cpm monocularly.
- If the patient has difficulty clearing −2.00 with MAF, it suggests accommodative insufficiency.
- If the patient has difficulty clearing +2.00 with MAF, it suggests accommodative excess.
- If the patient has difficulty clearing +2.00 and −2.00 with MAF, it suggests accommodative infacility.

Binocular Accommodative Range

Binocular accommodative range shows the amount by which accommodation can be binocularly relaxed and stimulated at a near-testing distance of 40 cm and still be able to maintain single, clear binocular vision. Positive relative accommodation (PRA) is the amount of accommodation in excess of the accommodation needed for convergence. It shows the ability of the patient to stimulate accommodation while converging at the near object. Minus lenses are added and to keep the target clear, the patient must stimulate his accommodation. Negative relative accommodation (NRA) is the amount of accommodation below that of convergence. This is another form of accommodative insufficiency which shows the amount by which accommodation can be binocularly relaxed at a near-testing distance of 40 cm and still be able to maintain single clear binocular vision. Plus lenses are added and to keep the target clear, the patient must relax his accommodation. NRA can also be used to determine whether a patient has been over-minused during subjective refraction. NRA test is done at 40 cm distance with distance correction at which a nonpresbyopic patient should accommodate approximately +2.50D to see the object clearly. Any finding greater than +2.50D will suggest that the patient is over-minused.

This is an indirect form to test binocular vision disorder. The primary objective is to determine whether the patient would be benefitted by near addition or not. In a nonpresbyopic patient, the two findings, i.e., NRA and PRA, should be fairly large and well centered, for example NRA = +2.50D and PRA = -2.50D. The test is started with plus lens. Plus lenses are inserted in 0.25D steps until the first sustained blur (NRA) is noticed and then minus lenses are inserted in 0.25D steps until the first sustained blur is noticed (PRA). Thus, it tests interaction between accommodation and vergence.

- A higher NRA value suggests that the patient will be benefitted by near addition because the focusing system tires after constant near work.
- A low NRA reveals accommodative spasticity, i.e., the patient is having accommodative excess. The patient will be benefitted by a continuing session of vision therapy.
- Reduced PRA and NRA suggest accommodative infacility.

Lag of Accommodation

Accommodative lag may be thought of as an inaccuracy of accommodative function. It measures the extent to which the accommodative response is less than the dioptric stimulus to accommodate. In a normal subject, it is common to have an accommodative lag of 0.50–0.75D. Most patients underaccommodate for the target, but some will overaccommodate. It defines the patient's accommodative posture. Clinically, it may be measured using the following tests:

- Monocular estimation method (MEM) retinoscopy **(Fig. 6.3)**
- Fused cross cylinder test.

Positive lens indicates positive accommodation lag and negative lens indicates negative accommodation lag. Typically, the accommodative response to a target is slightly less than the accommodative stimulus. A lag greater than +1.00D is often seen in the patients with accommodative insufficiency or infacility, suggesting the need for plus lens at near. A lag of -0.25D or more usually indicates accommodative excess.

The PRIO unit has been specifically designed for measuring the lag of accommodation. The front of the instrument simulates a computer screen, and the instrument has a hole in the middle through which the clinician can perform retinoscopy.

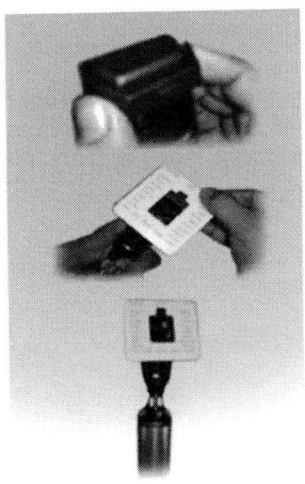

Fig. 6.3: Examples of MEM cards.

TREATMENT

The first line of treatment for any anomaly of accommodative function is correction of refractive error. Even a small amount of refractive error matters. A low plus lens in the range of +0.50D to +1.00D over the distance correction is very effective treatment. The computer user finds it very easy to work on a computer with a small amount of additional plus lens as he can work without having to use much of accommodation. This may blur his distance vision, but the amount of blur is usually tolerable to the patient in the office environment. So, it is prudent to demonstrate the distant blur and prescribe on the patient's response. In case the distance blur is not acceptable to the patient, a different glass in the form of occupational enhanced near vision or any other multifocal may be designed for him.

Vision therapy is very effective to increase the amplitude of accommodation and accommodative facility up to age-expected performance. An ideal vision therapy session for a given patient must include some in clinic activities followed by some home therapy processes. Computerized home therapy systems are available which can be installed on a patient's computer to enable him to work in his office or home.

Chapter 6: Accommodative Function and its Management

Multiple Choice Questions-Answers

1. The mechanism whereby the focusing ability of the eye is increased so that a distinct image of the object is maintained even when the object is brought nearer is called:
   a. Accommodation
   b. Aperture
   c. Retina control
   d. None of above

2. The muscles that control the shape of the lens are called:
   a. Ciliary muscles
   b. Tangential muscles
   c. Smooth muscles
   d. Lens muscles

3. Which of the following is not an important part of sequential management consideration for accommodative dysfunction?
   a. Correction of ametropia
   b. Added lenses
   c. Vision therapy
   d. Prism

Answer Key

| 1. | (a) | 2. | (a) | 3. | (d) |

Self-Practice Questions

1. What elements of Accommodative Function should be evaluated when a pre-presbyopic individual is complaining of computer-related vision problem?

2. Hrithik, a 22-year-old guy, presented with complaints of blurred vision and eyestrain after working on visual display unit (VDU) for 45 minutes to 1 hour. Although he reported similar symptoms during his college days, the problem had become worse since he joined his job as a software engineer. He was otherwise healthy and was not taking any medication. Suggest management.

CHAPTER 7

Binocular Vision and its Management

SYMPTOMS

A patient with a disorder in binocular vision function usually reports the following symptoms in common:
- He complains of eyestrain
- He complains of headache
- Blurring of reading object
- Diplopia
- Difficulty concentrating
- Loss of comprehension over time
- A pulling sensation
- Movement of the text on the screen
- Skipping lines/reading same lines
- Slow reading.

RATIONALE

Two eyes of the human being are located in two different sockets at a distance to each other. Each receives a little different signal from the same object which has to fuse together to see the object singly and clearly. The mechanism which is responsible for one single clear vision is known as binocular single vision. The two eyes have to work together as a team to provide sustained comfortable and clear single vision. In order to allow binocular vision, it is essential that both eyes are correctly aligned when viewing the object. The position of each eye in the orbit is controlled by extraocular muscles. A slight difference in the length, insertion, or strength of the same muscles in the two eyes can lead to the tendency for one eye to drift to a different position in its orbit from the other, resulting in phoria. This is quite common when there is a pressure of excessive visual demand. In many cases, the visual axes are slightly misaligned and similar images do not fall on the exact corresponding retinal points. The human visual system is capable to correct these small imperfections in alignment by way of the fusion mechanism. A constant neuromuscular effort is required to keep the eyes aligned. The eye alignment at near-viewing distance is more complex than at distance because of the interaction between the convergence and accommodative mechanism as happens in case of computer tasks. For a prolonged computer task, the desire for binocular single clear vision creates extra demand on the binocular vision system. According to Law 2 of the "Laws of Computer Vision," the elements of the visual system control the performance of visual skills. The ability of the function is adversely affected that deteriorates the performance of visual skills. The constant convergence on computer display deteriorates the ability, leading to visual deficiency. Law 4 of the "Laws of Computer Vision" says that a deficiency in any of the visual skills will lead to symptoms of CVS. The subject fatigues faster and performs below par.

TWO EYES—AS A PAIR

The two eyes work in synergy. However, in binocular vision, the two eyes do not affect the visual consciousness with equal force—one eye leads the other and performs the major function of seeing; the leading eye is called the dominant eye and the fellow eye is called the nondominant eye. While lining up two objects, the visual system relies more on the dominant eye, even though the nondominant eye is kept open. An approximate judgment of the alignment can be made binocularly, but the binocular projection center will usually be found to lie nearer the dominant eye.

The concept Ocular Dominance may be studied in three different categories—Sensory Dominance, Oculomotor Dominance, and Directional Dominance. Sensory Dominance may occur when the visual system finds it easier to suppress one eye and favors another eye because of the difference in image clarity, color, and brightness. Oculomotor dominance occurs when an eye does a better job of fixating centrally in the presence of fixation disparity. Directional dominance is the sighting dominance, i.e., the eye that is sighted at the target and leads the other eye in fixating at the target in binocular vision. The other eye is the nondominant eye that follows the dominant eye and looks at the same target slightly at a different angle. The small difference provides the required depth perception. It must be understood that ocular dominancy has nothing to do with the visual acuity.

The phenomenon of ocular dominance is clinically important in the study of binocular vision. Eye dominance has important implications for reading. In normal eye teaming, the dominant eye orchestrates the tracking of both eyes. The right eye naturally tracks from left to right while the left eye naturally tracks from right to left. People with left eye dominancy will initially want to look at the right side of the page first and then to move to the left, thus causing difficulties in reading languages that move from left to right like English.

The knowledge of an individual's ocular dominancy is also useful while considering the "monovision" approach to temporary or long-term unilateral refractive correction with contact lenses or surgery. The monovision technique was initially devised for the convenience of presbyopic contact lens wearers, but ocular surgery has embraced this approach in conjunction with intraocular lens implantation and refractive procedures with a high rate of success and a high degree of patient satisfaction. In monovision, the dominant eye is usually corrected for distance and the other eye is corrected for near vision (**Fig. 7.1**).

There are certain occupations, such as shooting, where a dominant eye can make hitting moving targets easier. People who practice photography can also benefit from a dominant eye. Refer to Chapter 4 where it has been explained that the location of the visual targets plays an important role in determining sitting posture for people working on a computer.

Eye dominancy is someone's innate characteristics. A stable dominant eye is very important to hold the visual system steady at the fixating target. If there is a dominancy conflict, then often attention jumps several words or lines and hence affects comprehension, leading to binocular instability. It is, therefore, important that natural eye dominancy is always maintained and not disturbed.

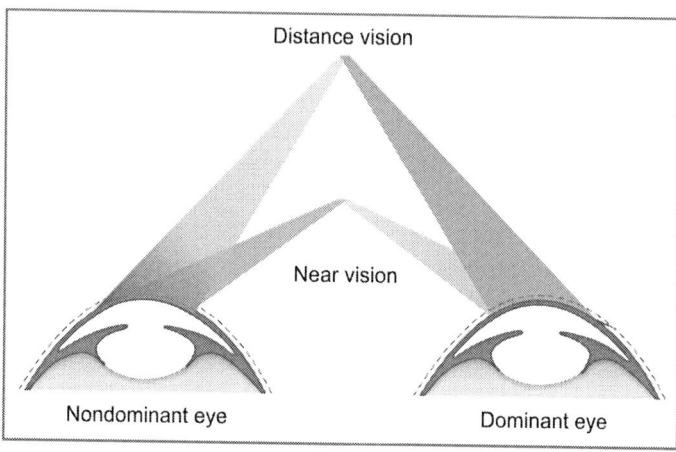

Fig. 7.1: Schematic representation of mono vision.

There are other advantages of having two eyes. The two eyes acuity taken together is better by approximately half a line of letters on the Snellen chart, compared with just one eye alone. The binocular visual field is also larger by nearly 30°, compared to monocular visual field. The most important advantage of binocular vision is a high degree of stereopsis. Stereopsis is one such attribute that evidently provides so much advantage to those who have it that it is often termed "barometer" of the binocular vision.

CLINICAL EXAMINATION OF BINOCULAR VISION

Studies have shown clinically significant esophoria and exophoria in the pre-presbyopic population of computer users. This is probably a reflection of high near-point demands of computer tasks. By convention, 40 cm is the standard distance at which the near vision is assessed. The computer monitor is usually at a distance of 50–60 cm, where the accommodative and convergence demand are somewhat less. A diagnosed binocular vision problem at 40 cm almost certainly indicates a binocular vision problem at a computer screen.

In order to do the complete evaluation of binocular vision function for a patient complaining of computer vision syndrome, the set of tests as shown in the **Flowchart 7.1** may be conducted.

Flowchart 7.1: Binocular vision function tests.

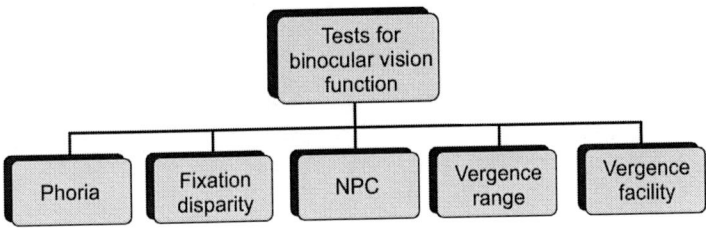

Phoria

When a person with normal binocular vision looks at an object, both visual axes converge such that they intersect at the object of regard. If the person is orthophoric, then only tonic vergence is responsible for turning each eye to the point at the target. When the phoria is present, both tonic vergence and fusional vergence are responsible for turning each eye at the target. When the amount of phoria is just enough to be corrected by fusional vergence reserve, it is called compensated phoria. If the phoria is so large that fusional vergence reserve cannot correct it, the phoria is referred to as a decompensated phoria. Fusional vergence represents the amount of convergence or divergence that can be induced to maintain fusion without changing accommodation. When the phoria is decompensated and the person looks at an object, only one visual axis points at the target and the other visual axis points away from the target in the direction determined by the type of phoria the person is afflicted with. Majority of cases of phoria are completely symptom-free or compensated; few may be symptomatic or decompensated. In such cases, difficulties may be severe with regard to binocularity. Exophoria is quite commonly noticed in a computer user. The tests for phoria are entry test for overall binocular vision assessment. The tests are conducted by breaking the fusion with dissimilar targets. When the fusion is broken by dissimilar visual targets, the eyes move to their natural resting position that may be eso, exo, hyper, or hypo. The tests are done at a distance of 6 m and also at 40 cm. The test at 40 cm distance is most relevant to the computer users. Both horizontal and vertical phoria should be measured. A small amount of exophoria is accepted. Esophoria with visually related symptoms

Chapter 7: Binocular Vision and its Management

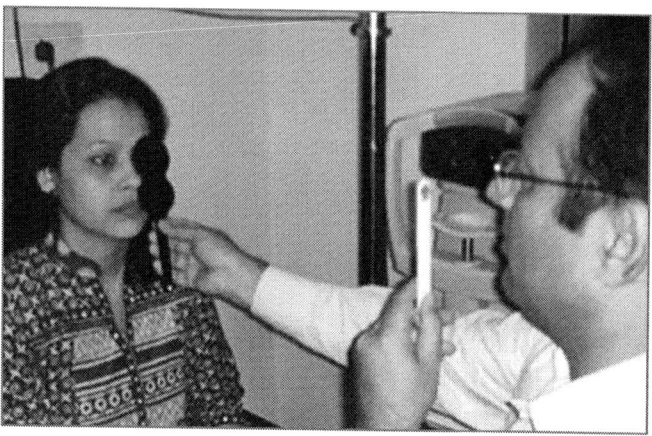

Fig. 7.2: Cover test.

should be suspected. A vertical phoria of 1.00D or even 0.50D may cause generalized asthenopic symptoms. The other symptoms may be disorientation or losing one's place while reading. The preferred methods for phoria measurement are:
- Cover test **(Fig. 7.2)**
- Howell phoria test
- Maddox rod test
- Von Graefe technique

Fixation Disparity

Fixation disparity evaluates the accuracy of the binocular vision system. Binocular vision is optimal when the fixated target is imaged onto the center of the fovea of each eye, so that the principal visual direction of both eyes intersects at the fixation point. However, even subjects who have normal binocular vision with good stereo acuity may have slight deviation from the optimal state. These small errors in alignment typically amount to a few minutes of arc and are called fixation disparity. Fixation disparity is not always considered abnormal. It is a physiological variant of normal binocular vision during which foveal fusion is maintained. It is slight manifest misalignment of visual axes which may be horizontal, vertical, or torsional. If the visual axes of both eyes cross at the point of regard, the subject does not have any fixation disparity, whereas if the visual axes cross before the point of regard, the subject indicates the presence of decompensated eso deviation, implying the presence of over-convergence. If the visual axes cross beyond the point of regard, the subject indicates the presence of decompensated exo deviation, implying the presence of under-convergence. This is how the presence of fixation disparity often indicates stress on fusional vergence, resulting in asthenopia, reduced depth perception, and reduced quality of binocular vision. The subject tends to suffer from visual fatigue during near work. For the computer workstation, it is relevant to know to what extent fixation disparity may depend on the position of the screen relative to the eyes as fixation disparity is strongly affected by the viewing distance. The presence of fixation disparity can be detected by Brock String **(Fig. 7.3)** and can be assessed clinically with the help of Mallet Test. The distance and near tests are performed separately with the Mallet unit. The Mallet unit measures the associated phoria which is the amount of prism that is needed, under binocular conditions of viewing to restore a fixation disparity position of the eyes to the ortho position. Dissociated phoria, on the other hand, is defined as a deviation from the orthovergence position that occurs when no fusional contours are provided. While "dissociated" refers to measurements

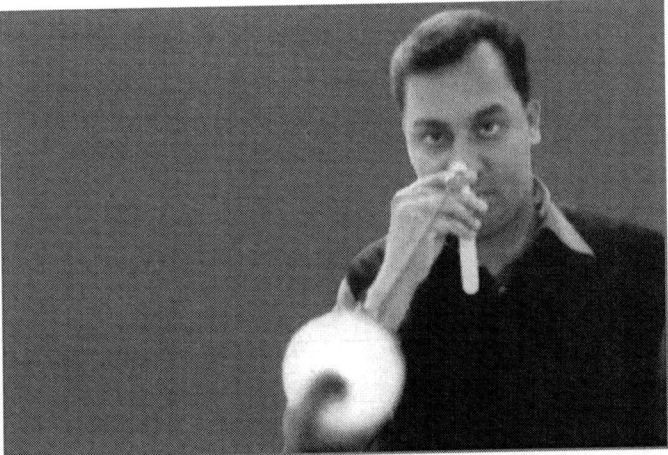

Fig. 7.3: Brock string.

under eliminated fusion, "associated" refers to measurements in the presence of fusion stimuli. The term associated phoria refers to the value of the prism that nulls a fixation disparity detected under conditions of partial dissociation. Fixation disparity and associated phoria have been thought to be an indicator of a decompensated phoria that gives rise to symptoms.

Vergence Range

Vergence function is assigned to the motor system of the eyes. They align the eyes in such a way that they ensure and maintain binocular fixation and binocular vision. Vergence range represents the amount of convergence or divergence that can be induced to maintain fusion without changing accommodation. The measurement of fusional vergence range is an important clinical test in the assessment of binocular vision status to know how much of total fusional vergence amplitude is required to correct the phoria. In general, the vergence range should be quite large and well centered for comfortable vision. Positive and negative fusional reserves are the two important clinical measurements used to assess the fusional vergence reserve. The ability to bring the eyes together is called "Positive Fusional Vergence" (PFV) and the ability to diverge the eyes is called "Negative Fusional Vergence" (NFV). The following tests are usually applied to measure PFV and NFV:
- Step Vergence Test
- Smooth Vergence Test

PFV and NFV can be measured at distance and near separately by placing appropriate prisms before the eyes until the fusion breaks down and diplopia results. The near test is more important for the computer workers.

Near Point of Convergence

Near point of convergence (NPC) is the test to assess the convergence amplitude. When an individual focuses on the near object, it is necessary for the eyes to turn inward toward each other. Therefore, a remote NPC is most frequently used as a criterion to diagnose convergence insufficiency.

The test should be applied on all patients with near-point symptoms. An NPC of smaller than 8 cm is to be suspected. However, even if the patient is able to converge to 2-3 cm, convergence insufficiency is not necessarily ruled out. Repeated measures of NPC result in a dramatic increase in the measure. Age has not been seen to have any impact on NPC.

Testing for NPC should start at a distance of 40 cm or 16 inches. It is performed by slowly moving a target toward the patient's eyes until the patient reports diplopia or the examiner notices a break in fusion. Target selection is an important issue for NPC test. The test should be performed with both accommodative and nonaccommodative targets. Many patients demonstrate obvious discomfort while crossing their eyes. For these patients, hold the target close to their NPC for 10 seconds and then ask if they feel any discomfort. A positive response confirms the diagnosis.

Vergence Facility

Vergence facility is the ability to quickly change where the eyes are pointing when looking between objects at different distances (Fig. 7.4). Under normal seeing condition, convergence occurs when the object approaches the eyes and divergence occurs when an object recedes. Vergence facility is the ability to rapidly and accurately fuse the two images from the two eyes from near to far and vice versa. The

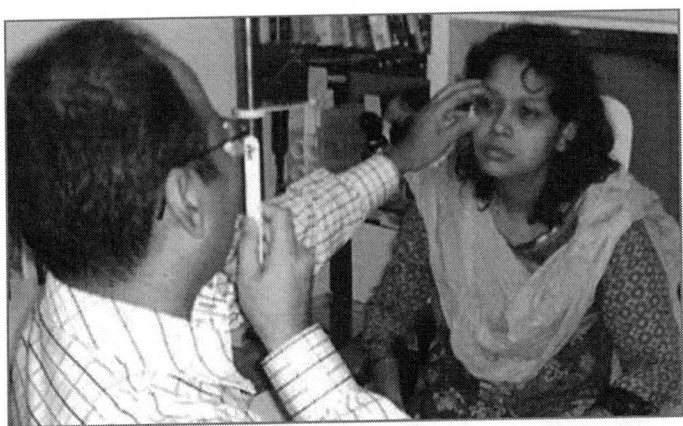

Fig. 7.4: Vergence facility test.

eyes work as a team to maintain the "oneness" in all directions of gaze. Any slowness or slackness in looking onto an object can lead to double vision and poor timing.

The test to measure vergence facility evaluates the stamina and dynamics of vergence response. This is the measure of the ability to make rapid repetitive vergence changes over an extended period of time. Another characteristic that we indirectly measure using vergence facility test is sustaining ability, i.e., the ability of an individual to maintain vergence at a particular level for a sustained period of time. Thus, it measures the dynamics of the fusional vergence system and the ability to respond over a period of time. This is a very important issue for the computer users who need to converge on the screen for a sustained period of time and also need to alter their vergence between keyboard and screen and to source document repetitively.

The vergence facility is measured with the help of a vergence facility prism combination of 12 base out and 3 base in. It is quite likely that a symptomatic patient may show normal fusional amplitude but a reduced vergence facility.

TREATMENT

The chief concern of the patients with computer vision syndrome is to overcome their symptoms or some visual performance deficiency. In any binocular, ocular motor, and accommodative dysfunction, the first management consideration is correction of a significant refractive error and then plan for the treatment of diagnosed binocular vision anomaly. Once the diagnosis of binocular vision anomalies is established, it is relatively easier to plan the sequence of treatment management. Lenses, prisms, mirrors, and vision training procedures are several options available to design the treatment plan. Lenses change accommodative and vergence demand, whereas prisms and mirrors change the direction of light. Plus lens induces base-in effect and minus lens induces base-out effect. The vision training program may be planned with various vision therapy tools such as Anaglyphs and Polaroid Filters, Septums, and Apertures and many other tools.

A high AC/A ratio suggest that a very large change in binocular alignment can be achieved with small addition of lenses. A low AC/A ratio indicates that the use of lenses will have little desirable effect. The use of lenses is, however, useful in some cases of a normal AC/A ratio.

In general, vertical phoria should be treated with the prism prescription. The most accepted criterion for determining the amount of vertical prism to prescribe is the associated phoria measurement, using fixation disparity test. In vertical heterophoria, prescribing the prism that reduces the fixation disparity to zero is the most ideal treatment. Exo deviations and convergence insufficiency are often seen together which can be best treated with vision therapy. Eso deviations are most successfully treated with plus lenses for near as they relax accommodative convergence. The plus prescription can be in single-vision glasses or in the multifocal form. Vision therapy may be an added successful treatment for such conditions. When both vertical and horizontal phoria are present, the clinician should first consider prism correction of the vertical component. Vertical prism may be helpful to decrease suppression and increase fusional ranges.

Multiple Choice Questions-Answers

1. **Which of the following is considered to be the entry point into the analysis of accommodative and binocular vision data for the primary care of binocular vision disorder?**
    a. Phoria for distance and near
    b. AC/A ratio
    c. Fixation disparity
    d. Lag of accommodation

2. **Which of the following is the primary contribution of binocularity to human visual perception?**
    a. Stereopsis
    b. Color discrimination
    c. Contrast
    d. Spatial localization

3. Which of the following is not true about prism?
   a. Prism can be used to increase or decrease the difficulties of the task
   b. Prism is useful to help the patient eliminate the suppression
   c. Prism is not used for accommodative dysfunction, unless there is an associated binocular problem
   d. Prism is used to improve the patient's ability to relax accommodation

Answer Key

| 1. | (a) | 2. | (a) | 3. | (d) |

Self-Practice Questions

1. Vergence range measurement norms, which were made for 40 cm test distance, may not apply to computer working distance. How can the clinician deal with this dilemma?
2. What is the difference between associated and dissociated phoria?
3. What are the attributes of binocularity to human visual perception? What happens when the binocularity is disturbed because of extravisual stress?

CHAPTER 8

Eye Movement Disorder and its Management

SYMPTOMS

Eye movement skills affect the reading ability of the computer user. If there is any compromise in any of the eye movement skills, the person may show one or more of the following symptoms:
- Loss of place while reading
- Re-reading words or lines of text
- Word omissions
- Skipping entire lines or reading words in the improper order
- Using compensatory method like finger or marker to keep place
- Overall reading speed is affected
- Asthenopia and generalized fatigue

It should also be remembered here that deficient language skills also cause reading disorders.

RATIONALE

Different types of eye movements are seen during reading. Eye movements are the results of action of the extraocular muscles. There are six extraocular muscles that are designed to stabilize and move the eyes. These muscles are:
1. Superior Rectus Muscles (SR)
2. Inferior Rectus Muscles (IR)
3. Medial Rectus Muscles (MR)
4. Lateral Rectus Muscles (LR)
5. Superior Oblique Muscles (SO)
6. Inferior Oblique Muscles (IO)

These muscles are attached to the globe by broad, flat, thin insertions and at the back of the eye in the Annulus of Zinn. The only muscle which is not attached in the annulus area is the inferior oblique which is attached nasally at the anterior floor of the orbit. The eyeball performs rotatory movements around the center of rotation which is a hypothetical point that lies approximately 13.5 mm behind the apex of the cornea when measured on line of sight (**Fig. 8.1**). During movements, certain muscles increase their activity while others decrease it. The action of the six extraocular muscles for eye movement depends on the position of the eye at the time of muscles' contraction. Horizontal eye movements are rather simple. Increased activity of the lateral rectus will direct the pupil laterally, while increased activity of the medial rectus will direct it medially. However, movements of the eyes above or below the horizontal plane are complicated and require, at the minimum, activation of pairs of muscles.

Extraocular muscles are striated skeletal muscles and like all other skeletal muscles, extraocular muscles are made of fibers. They are among the fastest muscles in the body. The speed and precision of extraocular muscles are unsurpassed anywhere in the body. Extraocular muscles are highly fatigue resistant, yet the mechanism involved in the fusion process is so highly complex that it may result in muscle fatigue, resulting into disruption of the fusion mechanism.

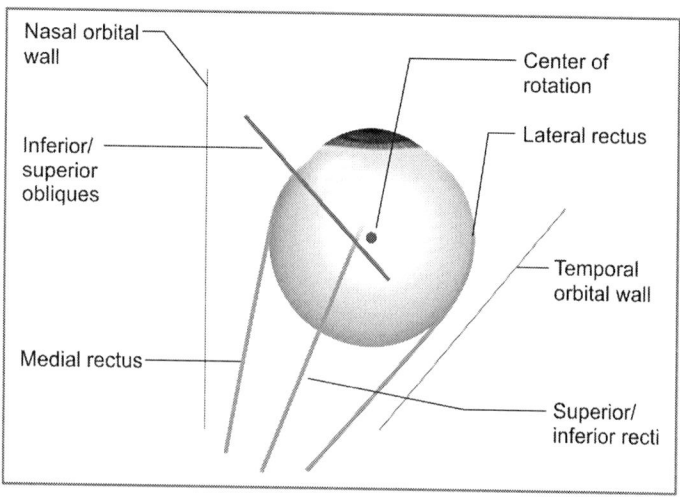

Fig. 8.1: Schematic view of right eye from the above.

Law 1 of "Laws of Computer Vision" says that the computer workers fixate at the target and then follow the same. Fixation and Depth perception are, therefore, primary visual skills for them. Saccades and Regressions are the two other important visual skills needed for reading task. Any disorder in any of the eye movement skills will adversely affect the functional capabilities of the computer user.

IMPORTANT EYE MOVEMENT SKILLS FOR READING

During reading, the three important components of eye movement are:
1. Fixation
2. Saccades
3. Regressions

Fixation

The term "fixation" is used to indicate the seemingly steady maintenance of the image of the object of regard on the fovea. It refers to the position maintenance and is due to combined involvement of saccades, pursuits, vestibular ocular reflexes, and vergences. For a normal reader, the average duration of fixation is 200-500 ms. The computer user fixates at the object of regard and then follows it. Reading difficulties and various other symptoms may occur with poor fixation ability because of inefficiency in any of the above functions.

Saccades

Saccades have been a diagnostic and management concern for the optometrists because of their importance in the act of reading. Saccades are fast eye movements with a fixational pause between two saccades. Saccades enable us to rapidly redirect our line of sight so that the point of interest stimulates the fovea. Average saccade is 8-9-character space which is about 2°. The ideal saccade is a single eye movement that rapidly reaches and abruptly stops at the target of interest. The velocity changes during its course, being faster at the beginning and slower at the end of the sweep. Saccades may be inaccurate in two ways. The most common inaccuracy is slight undershoot, i.e., the saccade is slightly short of the target. A less common inaccuracy is an overshoot of the target.

Regression

Regression is right-to-left eye movement and it occurs 10–20% of the time in skilled readers. Regression occurs when the reader overshoots the target or misinterprets the text or has difficulties understanding the texts.

The above discussion establishes the fact that the reading ability is the function of all eye movements. Any disorder that affects one of them will also affect the other in some way or the other. It is, therefore, difficult to find saccadic dysfunction in isolation of fixational or pursuit anomalies. Together, we can use the term "ocular motor dysfunction" to refer to the condition in which problems are present in all areas of eye movements. On the whole, poor eye movement skills can cause below-average reading ability. Reading process is also accompanied with processes such as attention, memory, and the utilization of the perceived visual information. It has been established that there is a relationship between poor ocular motor skills and attention deficit. According to law 4 of "laws of computer vision," if there is any deficiency in the ability of any of the elements of the visual system, it implies that visual demands exceed visual ability. It may lead to one or more symptoms of CVS. The deficient ocular motor function will most commonly show the following symptoms:

- Excessive head movement
- Frequent loss of place while reading
- Omission of words
- Skipping lines
- Slow reading speed
- Poor comprehension
- Short attention time
- Overall poor performance

Moreover, oculomotor dysfunctions are generally associated with accommodative, binocular, and visual perceptual dysfunctions. As a result, the treatment of eye movement disorder falls within the context of an overall treatment approach designed to deal with other problems as well. It is, therefore, important for the clinician to evaluate eye movement functions when an individual is complaining of computer vision syndrome.

CLINICAL EXAMINATION OF OCULAR MOTOR DYSFUNCTION

The ocular motor abnormalities are also associated with some serious etiologies. They are also susceptible to a large variety of medications. It is, therefore, important to take history regarding the onset and intake of medications. However, patients with symptoms of CVS mostly complain of functional difficulties that are associated with ocular motor dysfunction with no significant underlying pathology. The functional ocular motor disorder may affect the efficiency of the individual working on a computer for longer hours. History is equally important to diagnose the functional disorder of ocular motor dysfunction. Those patients usually have a history of skipping lines and words while reading, loss of place while reading, poor comprehension, and slow reading speed. Besides, history taking objective observation can provide a fairly good idea to diagnose ocular motor dysfunction.

In order to assess the fixating ability of the eye, ask the patient to fixate monocularly on a given target and observe the steadiness of the eye. No noticeable drifting or eye movement should be present. If the patient is unable to maintain steady fixation, ask him to hold his thumb at 40 cm to determine if the proprioceptive input from the "hand support" is of any help in maintaining steady eye positioning. Sometimes, the problem may be psychological, i.e., lack of attention or fatigue. In such case, it is very much possible to plan treatment through appropriate environmental changes and vision training procedure.

General observation of eye movement can be done with the patient sitting and being asked to follow the fixation stick. The practitioner moves the stick smoothly in a figure of eight and the patient follows. While the patient follows the stick, the practitioner observes his eye movement that should correspond to the stick all through the loop. If any jerk is noted, tracking skill is suspected. Saccades can be assessed as shown in **Figure 8.2**. The patient looks at the red or green stick on call from the practitioner. Any overshooting or undershooting is recorded.

TREATMENT

The treatment of functional ocular motor dysfunction is based on the assumption that the problems and difficulties are present in all areas. It

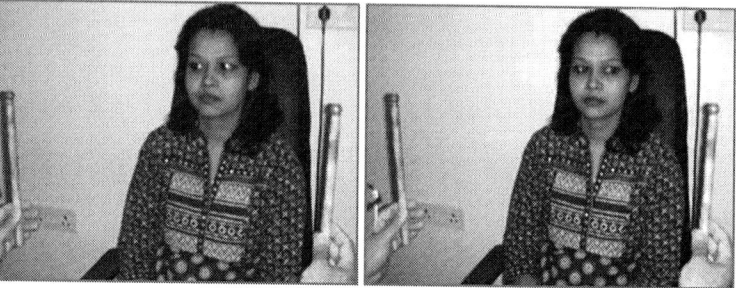

Fig. 8.2: Saccadic eye movement.

forms the part of the overall treatment of the binocular vision disorder. Like any other treatment for binocular vision disorder, prescribing for any uncorrected refractive error is the first consideration. Accurate fixation, saccades, and pursuits highly depend on optimal visual acuity. Prisms have no role in the treatment of functional ocular motor dysfunction. Added lenses may be helpful if there are associated accommodative and binocular problems that warrant the use. Vision therapy treatment plan is designed for the overall condition and not just for saccades and pursuits. This is because it is important to simulate natural seeing conditions in the therapy program, and all procedures require precise fixational skills.

Multiple Choice Questions-Answers

1. **Human eye movement of back and forth during the reading process in inquiry is defined as:**
   a. Saccades
   b. Fixation
   c. Pursuits
   d. Regressions

2. **Which of the following extraocular muscles (EOMs) is not attached to the globe in Annulus of Zinn?**
   a. IO
   b. IR
   c. SO
   d. SR

Chapter 8: Eye Movement Disorder and its Management

3. Which of the following is not true about saccades?
   a. Saccades are fast eye movement
   b. Saccades shift the fixation abruptly
   c. Saccades redirect the line of sight so that the point of interest stimulates the fovea
   d. Saccades allow us to follow the moving object

Answer Key

| 1. | (d) | 2. | (a) | 3. | (d) |

Self-Practice Questions

1. Eye movement disorders are rarely present in isolation. They are usually found associated with accommodative, binocular, and visual perceptual dysfunctions. Explain with reference to symptoms of computer vision syndrome.

2. Explain the tests that can be used to diagnose the ocular movement disorder.

CHAPTER 9

Computer Use and Dry Eye

SYMPTOMS

Dry eye is a chronic, symptomatic, ocular surface disease. The condition is multifactorial, characterized by impairment of the integrity of tear film and cornea that affects visual functions in a limited manner. Experiencing dry eye symptoms can be debilitating for the subject who would invariably present the following symptoms:
- He complains of burning sensation in the eyes.
- He feels gritty or sand particle-like feeling in the eyes.
- He feels the presence of foreign body-like feeling in the eyes.
- Irritations in the form of itching
- Redness of the eye
- Sensitivity to light
- He complains of blurred vision that improves on blinking.
- Excess watering of the eye
- Mucus discharge from the eyes.

RATIONALE

The tear film is a very thin layer over the ocular surface. A deficiency in either the quantity or the quality of the tear film can lead to dry eyes. Broadly speaking, there are two reasons for dry eye symptoms as shown in **Flowchart 9.1**.

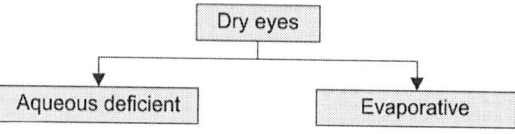

Flowchart 9.1: Dry eyes—causes.

Both the types of dry eyes lead to decreased tear film stability. Evaporative-type dry eyes are more common in a computer user. However, both types occur simultaneously in the most severe cases. Evaporative-type dry eyes can be related to multiple clinical signs, the most common among them being as follows:
- Meibomian oil deficiency
- Lid aperture disorders
- Low blink rate
- Ocular surface allergy
- Reduced tear breakup time (TBUT)
- Reduced tear meniscus height

Law 3 of "Laws of Computer Vision" says that visual postures are influenced by visual environment. Computer users experience dry eyes symptoms because of unique visual posture that features a higher viewing angle, larger palpebral aperture, and lower workplace humidity together with a decreased blink rate. Dry eye disturbs the natural function and protective mechanisms of the external eye that lead to an unstable tear film during the open eye state. Sometimes, the condition worsens and disturbs the quality of life **(Fig. 9.1)**.

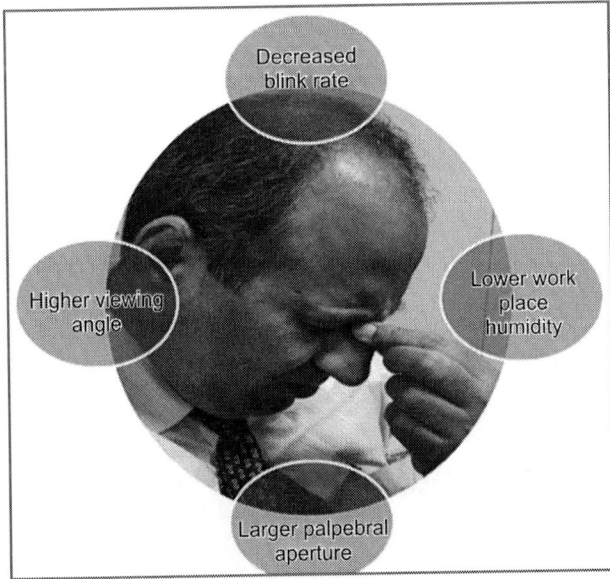

Fig. 9.1: Dry eyes disturb quality of life.

Decreased Blink Rate

The computer user while working on a computer hardly blinks more than 4-6 times per minute. This is much less than the normal blink rate of 15 blinks per minute. This is a clear indication to support the facts that the blink rate decreases during the computer use. Possible explanation for the decreased blink rate may include concentration on the task or a relatively limited range of eye movement. Regular blinking is necessary to properly re-form the tear layer on a regular basis. The decreased blink rate coupled with an increased rate of tear evaporation occurs with most computer workers and they experience ocular drying while working at the computer.

Higher Viewing Angle

Computer work usually requires a higher gaze angle. A higher gaze angle results in a greater percentage of blinks that are incomplete, and incomplete blinks do not count. The reasons are simple. The tear lipids normally pool along the lower lid margin, and during a full blink the upper eyelids grab the lipids and spread them over the aqueous tear layer to form an oily layer of the tears. An incomplete blink does not allow this to occur; therefore, the evaporation of tears is more that results in loss of tear aqueous **(Fig. 9.2)**.

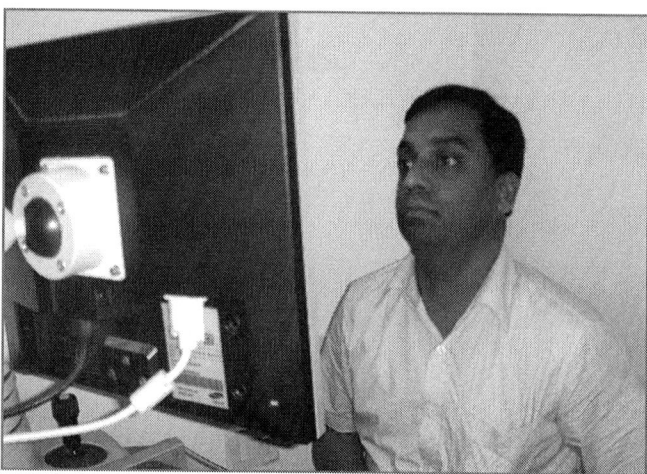

Fig. 9.2: Higher ocular gaze.

Larger Palpebral Aperture

The size of ocular aperture is related to the gaze elevation—as we gaze higher, our eyes are open wider **(Fig. 9.3)**. Studies have shown that an average exposed ocular surface is nearer to double while working on a computer than most other tasks. This causes tears' elimination through evaporation.

Lower Workplace Humidity

The office air environment is often low in humidity and may also contain contaminants. Relatively low humidity may cause drying of the skin, mucous membranes, and conjunctivae. Dryness of eye may lead to tearing and pain, especially in those wearing contact lenses and who work on computers. The symptoms increase in severity with time.

DIAGNOSIS OF DRY EYES

Computer-related dry eye condition can be easily diagnosed by history taking. Most of the symptoms that the computer user presents point toward the presence of dry eyes. However, the following clinical tests may establish the diagnosis:

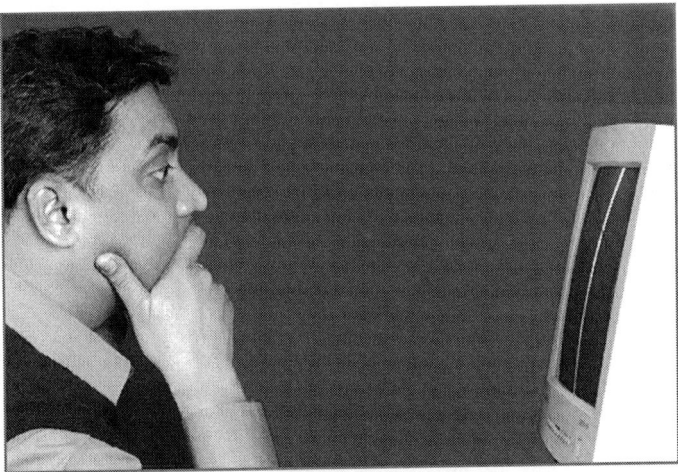

Fig. 9.3: Larger opening of the eyes.

Schirmer's Test

Schirmer's test measures the tear volume **(Fig. 9.4)**. It uses filter strips that are inserted behind the lower eyelids near the outer canthus area. The most acceptable point to insert the strip on the lower eyelid is the point that is two third from the nasal canthus and one-third from the temporal canthus. In both the eyes, strips are put together. The patient is asked to sit in an area which is away from direct light and direct air blows and is also asked to look straight ahead. Care must be taken not to touch the cornea while putting the strip. The strip moistens due to tear secretion. Roughly 15 mm of moisture in young and 10 mm of moisture in an old patient are taken as normal values. A patient with Sjogren's syndrome moistens <5 mm in 5 minutes. Sometimes, anesthetic drops are instilled into the eyes before putting up the strips to prevent tearing due to irritation from the paper itself. The test measures the basal tear secretion.

Tear Meniscus Height

The height and width of tear reservoir across the lower lid margin can give a reasonable assessment of tear volume. Use slit lamp and reduce the height of slit beam and adjust to the horizontal position.

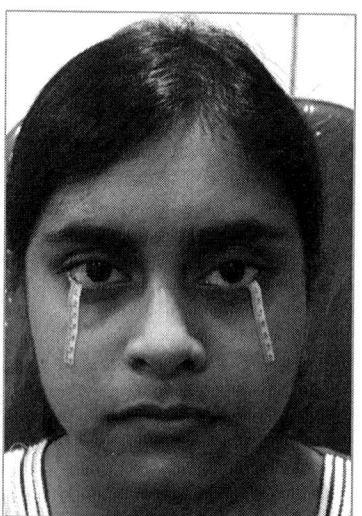

Fig. 9.4: Schirmer's test.

The approximate height of tear prism at the center in case of normal tear film is 0.2–0.4 mm and 0.2 mm at the periphery. Reduced height suggests reduced tear volume and increased height suggests a poor drainage system. Thin tear prism and/or scalloped edges of tear lake suggest poor tear quality.

Direct observation of the tears can provide indications as to the quality of the tears, i.e., good tears generally flow briskly with blink and contain few contaminants. Debris observed in tear meniscus is at times seen in dry eyes.

Tear Breakup Time Test

The TBUT test is then done to measure the stability of tears in the eyes, i.e., the time it takes for the tear to break up in the eye (**Fig. 9.5**). The test is done as follows:

Tears are stained with fluorescein dye and the lids are held wide apart with the help of hand. The time interval is measured between a complete blink and the first appearance of dry spot in the precorneal tear film using a slit lamp with cobalt blue light. The patient is not supposed to blink till then. The tear film breakup time must be at least 10 seconds. TBUT shorter than this can result in surface damage and very short TBUT (<2 minutes) indicates Keratoconjunctivitis sicca.

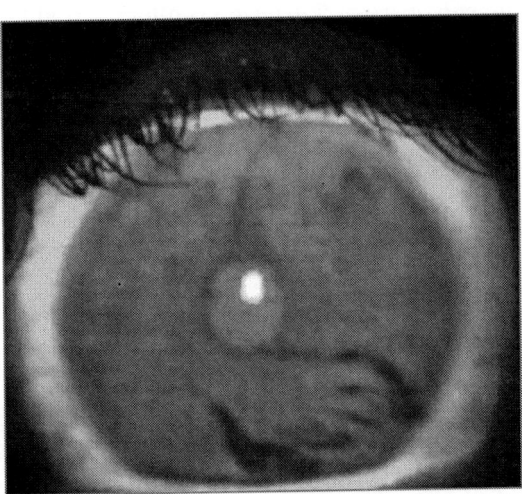

Fig. 9.5: Tear breakup time test.

Tear Thinning Time (TTT)

A keratometer is used instead of a slit lamp or a Tearscope. While the blink is held, the keratometer's mire images are observed and the time of the first disturbance is noted. Any image disturbance is attributed to alterations of the tear film. Shorter times than BUT have been reported, suggesting a greater sensitivity to tear film changes.

In addition, there are other tests like Rose Bengal Staining tests in which devitalized (sick) cells on the cornea, conjunctiva, and mucus in the tear film are detected using 1% Rose Bengal or 1% Lissamine green liquid or wetted strip. Lipid-Layer Thickness Assessment in which different patterns like color fringes, amorphous, flow pattern, or open meshwork may be observed is an indicator of lipid layer thickness.

MANAGEMENT

The increasing prevalence of dry eye due to increasing usage of computer, air pollution, and low humidity can easily be managed to relieve the symptoms. The following sequential steps may be followed:

Consider the Ergonomics of the Computer Workstation

The computer screen should be placed so that the worker is looking downward by 10-15°. The top of the screen should be below the eye level. If the patient is working near a window or ventilation, change of workstation position may be advised to change the airflow pattern. If possible, using a humidifier at the working station may help to minimize the effect of low humidity.

Patient Counseling

The patient should be educated that his condition is chronic and may have many additional contributing factors. So in order to minimize the effect of other associated factors:
- Avoid smoking,
- Reduce caffeine intake,
- Increase the amount of water he drinks—keeping a glass of water right in front of the computer screen will remind him to drink water which will also ensure a break and blink.
- He may be asked to consult his physician to alter the medications that could be aggravating the dry eye symptoms.

- The patient may be advised to blink more frequently and completely, especially when he begins to notice the symptoms.
- He may also be advised to take an occasional 2-minute break, look into the distance, and concentrate on blinking.

Treatment of Ocular Conditions

Treatment depends on the severity of the disease. A general stepwise approach should be used in the treatment of patients with dysfunction of the tear film. Tear replacement should be the first step and can be done with artificial tears that exist in many pharmaceutical presentations with or without preservatives. Some aqueous solutions containing polymers or macromolecules are used as tear substitutes. These increase the aqueous retention time and aqueous adherence to the ocular surface. Unfortunately, this replacement does not replace all biological properties and functions of the tear film, and these agents are especially useful for patients of a mild to moderate case. Treat the complicating ocular conditions such as blepharitis, meibomitis, and any other lid abnormalities. Blepharitis can be treated with lid scrubs or antibiotics or both. Meibomitis is treated with hot compresses and with lid hygiene.

Multiple Choice Questions-Answers

1. **What causes dry eyes for patients complaining of symptoms of computer vision syndrome?**
    a. Inadequate blinking
    b. Environment
    c. Medication
    d. All of the above

2. **Which of the following is one of the most common symptoms of dry eyes?**
    a. Headache
    b. Loss of peripheral vision
    c. Light sensitivity
    d. Floaters

3. Which of the following is one of the important natural ways to manage eye dryness?
   a. Avoid smoking
   b. Drink of plenty of water
   c. Wear sunglasses
   d. All of the above

Answer Key

| 1. | (d) | 2. | (c) | 3. | (d) |

Self-Practice Questions

1. What are the main causes of dry eyes for patients who are complaining of computer vision syndrome?
2. Design a suitable treatment regimen to alleviate dry eye symptoms related to computer use.

CHAPTER 10

Issues Related to Glare and Reflection

GLARE

Glare is a visual sensation that occurs because of excessive and uncontrolled lights or brightness. Not all people are equally sensitive to glare. Some are more sensitive and some are less sensitive. Age also affects glare sensitivity. In general, older people are more sensitive than younger people. The most common condition for glare is driving in the night when the illumination in a part of the visual field is much greater than the illumination to which retina is adapted. While working on computers, glare occurs when the level of illumination of the screen exceeds the level of illumination of the background, too much of light in the workplace, unequal or poor distribution of light and reflection of light from adjacent polished surfaces. Glare forms a veil of luminance which reduces the contrast, and thus the visibility of a target is decreased.

There are two types of glare as shown in **Flowchart 10.1**.

Discomfort Glare

Discomfort glare refers to the sensation one experiences when there is too bright overall illumination or reflection of light from adjacent polished surfaces or bright computer screen. A person is at a greater risk for experiencing discomfort glare when the light source is closer

Flowchart 10.1: Types of glare.

```
           Types of glare
           /           \
  Discomfort glare   Disability glare
```

to the fixation point. Computer users usually suffer from discomfort glare because horizontal gaze brings the light source closer to eyes and illuminated target creates difference in the illumination level in the visual field.

Disability Glare

Disability glare refers to the reduced visibility of a target due to light scatter within the globe by the ocular media. This scattered light forms a veil of luminance which reduces the contrast and thus the visibility of the target is reduced. It is basically caused by cataract, keratoconus, corneal edema, vitreous opacities, etc.

While it is true that our visual performance improves with light level, it is also not always true that more light is better. Computers are self-illuminating and require a different lighting arrangement. While the illumination produced by the lighting system may be ideal for paper tasks, it could create conditions that are absolutely dreadful for computer-based tasks. With paper tasks and typing, we look downward whereas while working on computers, we tend to look straight ahead at the screen. This leads to increase in glare caused by overhead lighting in our field of view either directly or in the periphery. Looking straight at our task, we also tend to see light that bounces off highly polished objects, such as picture frames, furnishings, mirrors, glass, and high-reflective wall surfaces.

Effects of Glare on Visual Performance of Computer Worker

The largest single enemy today in the workplace is the glare that may be defined as "light pollution" and the effect of which increases with the time spent **(Flowchart 10.2)**. Some of the common problems are:
- Contrast discrimination is an important ability to read and work faster and more accurately. Overhead lights or lights from window

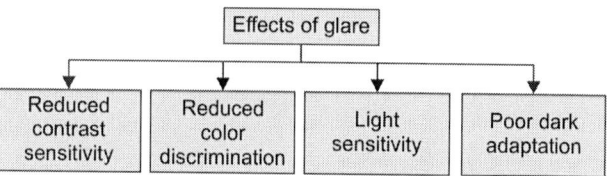

Flowchart 10.2: Effects of glare.

when they strike the illuminated objects on the computer monitor create light pollution in the viewing zone of the user which ultimately conflicts with the displays on the screen **(Fig. 10.1)**, thereby reducing the contrast.
- Color discrimination is an important attribute to work more efficiently on computers. The excessive luminance level creates a veiling effect on the computer display and thus creates a washed-out effect **(Fig. 10.2)**. This results in more difficulties to discriminate the colors. This is because of the adverse effect of a washed-out image on the retina.
- Discomfort glare also causes light sensitivity. The computer worker is horizontally looking in the room, as the screen is most of the time at the eye level. Bright open windows also pose the same risk as overhead light fixtures. A person is at a greater risk of experiencing discomfort glare when the source of light has a higher luminance and when it is closer to the point of attention. Some of the common symptoms of light sensitivity are rapid blinking, poor concentration, lowering of chin to shield the eyes, narrowing of the palpebral aperture, and epiphora.
- Light/dark adaptation is another problem that occurs because of glare present in the viewing field. This is because of large disparities in the brightness of objects in the field of view that occurs when viewing from brighter objects to darker objects or vice versa. The eye takes a brief period of time after the eye movement to adapt to the new brightness level. This is similar to what is noticed while

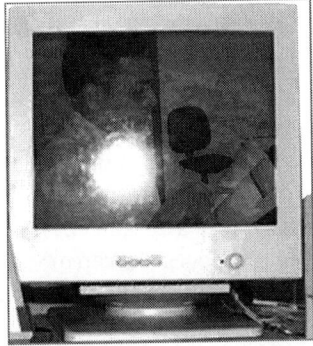

Fig. 10.1: Glare from overhead light source.

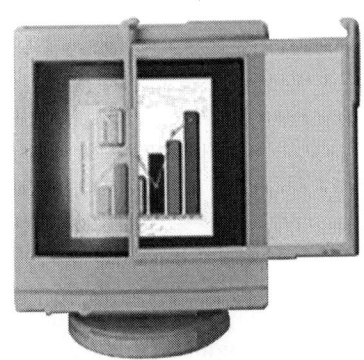

Fig. 10.2: Monitor with glare screen.

entering or leaving a dark movie theater. A similar effect occurs on a smaller scale when the eye needs to fixate back and forth from bright to dark objects in an office environment. When the eye is not properly adapted to the brightness level in which it is working, the vision is not good. This is a particular problem when constantly looking back and forth from a dark background computer display to a bright white reference document. If this process continues day by day, you are on road to first step toward macular degeneration.

Law 3 of "Laws of Computer Vision" states that visual abilities determine visual postures which will also be influenced by visual environment. Discomfort glare produces light pollution in the visual environment that influences the visual abilities of the computer user. In fact, computer vision syndrome is the by-product of compromised visual environment. The elimination of glare ensures visual hygiene and provides tranquil effect for eyes, improving visual performance and reducing the symptoms.

Checking the Presence of Glare

There is no standardized method available to check whether the glare is present or not or, in other words, the patient is having the problem of discomfort glare. However, we may design some practical methods based upon knowledge about the sources of the discomfort glare. The chief sources of Discomfort Glare are overhead lights, windows, reflective sources, and the computer screen itself. It is also a kind of overillumination. The following techniques may be applied to assess the effect of glare and relate to the source:

- Use a luminance meter to assess the amount of luminance; in this way, we can assess the overillumination.
- Dark and bright light in the viewing area also causes glare. Using the luminance meter, we can assess the luminance level around the objects in the field of view which can be differentiated from the luminance of the surrounding areas.
- The bright light from the peripheral vision creates nuisance. Ask the computer user to use his hands to shield the eyes like cap or visor and if he senses an immediate improvement in comfort, then we can diagnose that the worker is experiencing the discomfort glare. If the glare is from window, then shield the eyes from window. The test may be repeated twice or thrice to be sure about the diagnosis.

Flowchart 10.3: Sequential management considerations for glare.

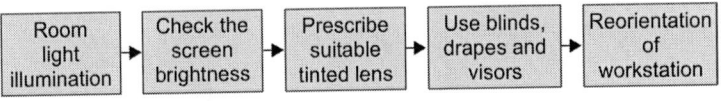

Solutions to Discomfort Glare

If the bright light contributes to discomfort, then it should be removed or mitigated in some manner. The following solutions may be tried sequentially as shown in **Flowchart 10.3**.

- A good lighting arrangement illuminates all of the visual objects in the field of view with nearly equal brightness. Overillumination, unequal distribution of illumination, improper light fitting, and auxiliary light fitting, all may cause discomfort glare. When you find out the source of discomfort glare, simply turn off the offending light source. Many a times, it is one single offending fixture in the ceiling that is creating nuisance.
- In the second step, check the screen brightness; the brightness of the screen should be adjusted to match the brightness of the visual objects that immediately surround it. Black letters on a white background are a better option than white letters on a black background.
- Tinted lenses per se do not help controlling the glare. The reasons are simple. Tinted lenses reduce light transmission and thereby reduce the overall effect of illumination. There are certain additional advantages of using tinted lenses as they increase contrast and reading comfort and provide relief to light-sensitive patients.
- Using blinds and drapes (**Fig. 10.3**) may be advised if the window view is considerably brighter than objects in the room; in such a case, it is wise to use blinds or drapes on windows. Using visor at times is also a very efficient way to eliminate the brightness of overhead fixtures.
- Reorientation of workstation may not be possible in many cases; hence, it should be considered at the last. It is aimed to eliminate the sources of bright light from the field of view. Sometimes, by just rotating the working desk by 90° so that light sources and bright window are not in the field of view works wonderfully. The idea is to control the brightness ratio of the screen to the window or light

96 Chapter 10: Issues Related to Glare and Reflection

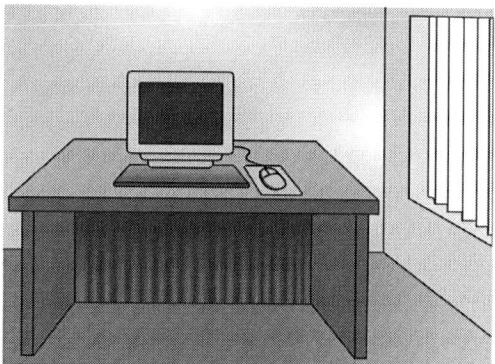

Fig. 10.3: Blinds are on the windows and the monitor is placed at an angle (perpendicular).

source. Windows are not the source of discomfort glare in large offices. In large modern offices, polished floorings, glass partitions, and polished tabletops may be the common sources of glare.

REFLECTION

Reflection of light causes loss of light transmission and creates a veiling effect, resulting in degradation of visual image. Trying to read a degraded image can certainly contribute to eyestrain or other visual discomfort. It is just like when the sky is reflected in a lake, the objects in the water are not seen. The reflections have the following negative effects:
- They reduce the contrast of the displayed visual information by adding reflected luminance to the emitted luminance.
- Reflected white light reduces the saturation of displayed colors.
- The image of light sources reflected in the screen causes the human visual system to focus on that image which is much degraded than the information shown on the screen. This makes focusing a stressful task which may cause headache and other severe disturbances.

Reflection and Computer Display

The old CRT screen had a lot of reflection issues, which have been mitigated to a great extent with the introduction of LCD and LED screens. Screen reflections are more noticeable when the person is using a dark background display, i.e., white characters on a black background. The reduction of contrast is noticed more with this polarity because of a darker background compared to the surrounding luminance. Switching over from dark background polarity to light background polarity may significantly reduce the reflection problem. In case the user cannot alter the polarity which is quite likely in many cases of ocular pathology, use of an Antireflection Filter may be indicated. The use of an Antireflection-Coated Filter is very useful for screens with a dark background in the presence of screen reflections. The reflection problem can also be mitigated by adjusting the screen brightness with the help of the brightness adjustment range of a computer display itself in case of a white background. Another way to prevent reflection is to put a hood on the computer display to stop light from impinging on it. This is like placing a visor over the screen. But it is not very effective as it completely blocks light and allows light only from selective directions.

Checking the Presence of Reflection

Most people are normally unaware of the screen reflections. The situation is somewhat similar to that of products displayed in the glass display window. They are so much occupied in seeing the product that they overlook the fact that the glass cover degrades the product visibility because of reflections. However, as a part of computer vision syndrome management process, the presence of reflections may be assessed in the patient's office environment.

Ask the patient to switch off his computer display and observe any mirror-like reflection on the screen. Then ask him to switch on the display. If the reflections degrade the visibility of the characters on the screen, you diagnose the presence of reflections. Now, you may try and find out the source by switching off the different lights in a sequential order.

Management

An optometrist can only suggest the remedial measures for reflection-related issues if he himself conducts a workplace evaluation. The following suggestions may help:
- Remove the source of the reflections, if possible. Use window blinds or turn off the offending lamp.

- Tilt or rotate the display to some other direction.
- Alter the workstation orientation to eliminate specular reflection.
- Replace the computer monitor if it is too old and scratched.
- Switch the polarity to dark characters on a light background.

ROLE OF ANTIREFLECTION COATED LENSES

Three phenomena occur when light strikes to an optical medium:
1. Reflection
2. Refraction, and
3. Absorption.

Light reflection occurs when rays of light bounce off the lens surface and change direction. The amount of light reflected depends upon lens material, lens curvature, or surface regularity. The reflection of light reduces light transmission and thus affects vision clarity. The higher the refractive index, the greater is the reflection. Reflection values for 1.50 index materials are typically 8%, 10% for 1.60 index materials, and 13% for 1.70 index materials. A curved surface produces less reflection than a flat surface. This is because parallel light beams, when they strike the flat surface, produce parallel reflected beams, even though they strike at different points on the surface. But when the lens surface is curved, the reflected rays will not be parallel. At each point on the surface, the law of reflection will apply, i.e., angle of incidence equals angle of reflection. The normal to the surface differs at each point on the curved surface. Dirt and defects on the lens surface further add to the reflection woes.

Glare is another issue. The computer users are more susceptible to glare because of their visual environment. Among the environmental factors the most important factor responsible for glare is illumination in the workplace. There are three sub-factors:
a. Intensity of illumination
b. Distribution of illumination
c. Quality of illumination.

Too much of light in workplace causes blinding glare. The bright light after striking the surrounding polished surface reflects and oscillates all around and enters the eyes together with the direct light, thus increases the quantity of light entering into the eyes.

Blinding glare not only makes vision more difficult by reducing the retinal sensitivity but is also physically painful. The pain is partly due to sustained maximal pupillary contraction. The impact is further increased because of the self-illuminated target and user's own visual posture.

Recent developments in computer screens, have, however, mitigated the glaring effect caused by computer screens. But reflection from surrounding visual environment still remains the matter of concern which is aggravated because of close proximity to light, wide open eyes and resultant dry eyes.

The distribution of light is the second important factor. Too much light in the peripheral field of view as often seen in workplace lowers the visual efficiency by reducing acuity and perpetuating after-images and thus causing distress. A balanced distribution of light in the background and surrounding environment is therefore, important to avoid glare and ensure comfort and efficiency.

The quality or the type of illumination is also an important factor. Natural light is generally accepted to be the best for psychological point of view which is rare in the workplace. As far as artificial lights are concerned the visual efficiency is better in white light and visual fatigue has been seen to appear more readily happening in yellow light.

Anti-reflection coating is applied to the lens surface to increase the light transmission through the lenses by minimizing the loss of light because of reflection from the lens surface. It means that anti-reflection coating per se may not provide a very effective solution to minimize the effect of glare for all computer users.

The most basic method that appears feasible for reducing the effect of glare is to reduce light illumination or light transmission to the eyes. While cutting down the light illumination in the entire workplace may not be possible in many cases, it can be effectively achieved in one of two ways: either excessive lights are being absorbed or reflected. Tinted lenses can be effectively used to absorb light and thereby reduce light transmission. Tints may be made to vary in density to tone down their effect of too much light absorption. They can also be effectively used by varying the tint density in different portions of the lens; for example, the top portion of the lens may be tinted, which may be further toned down to clear at the bottom. The author has successfully dispensed light pink indoor tint lenses with back surface anti-reflection coatings to many of his patients. Another method of dealing with light transmission may be the use of reflecting coatings on the front surface of the lens together with a back surface anti-reflection coating. This can be achieved by depositing layers of metal oxides of extreme thinness so that they remain transparent to a larger extent to luminous rays.

It is, therefore, not incorrect to conclude that, while anti-reflection coated lenses are useful when an individual has refractive error and must be used in all corrective lenses to see clearly, the use of plano anti-reflection lenses as a tool to prevent glare while working on digital devices when there is no need to wear correction because of the absence of refractive error, does not appear to be very useful.

Not to forget that reducing surface reflection also results in more visible dirt and defects on the lens. This may lead to difficulties in keeping the lens surface clean.

Nevertheless, anti-reflection coating is a wonderful attribute of modern lenses, and it should always be considered in most cases because of its usefulness to users.

ROLE OF BLUE CUT LENSES

Recently Blue Cut lenses, based upon the principle of selective light transmission have been introduced to protect the eyes from the high energy visible blue light. Blue light emitted from digital devices have been considered as one of the main reasons for digital eye strain.

The blue light has a very short, high energy wave. It is located at between 380 and 510 nm. It includes violets, indigo-blue and cyan **(Fig. 10.4)**. Sources of blue light include the sun, digital screens like TVs, computers, laptops, smart phones and tablets, electronic devices, and fluorescent and LED lighting.

Blue light is being considered as the main reason of digital eye strain. This is because people today spend too much time using digital gadgets at a close distance. Using digital devices up close or for long periods can lead to digital eye strain. The term digital eye strain in fact means different to different people. But in general eye strain is

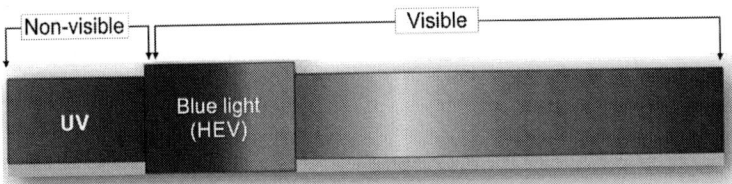

Fig. 10.4: Electromagnetic spectrum.

related to the intraocular and extraocular muscles of the eyes. Eye strain occurs when eye muscles get tired from intense use. Eye strain may occur because of any of the following factors:
- Long distance driving
- Constantly staring at computer screens
- Reading for a long time without pause
- Any activity that needs long sustained focusing
- Reading in dim light.

The manifestation of eye strain depends:
- Partly on the use to which the eyes are put
- Partly to the efficiency of the visual apparatus and
- Partly on the capacity of the individual to withstand sustained efforts.

Since blue light has short wavelength, they scatters more easily than most other visible light and causes glaring effect. This may make it difficult for your eyes to focus when receiving blue light. The contrast is reduced. The person finds it difficult to process blue light. Long exposure to blue light causes visual fatigue and near sightedness.

Numerous studies have shown that blue light regulates circadian rhythm and promote alertness, memory and cognition. The circadian rhythm synchronizes certain behavioural and biological processes through a daily cycle, partly regulated by sunlight. The processes that the circadian rhythm regulates include sleep-wake behaviour, hormone secretion, and cellular function. During the day the circadian system responds to the blue wavelengths of visible spectrum by releasing serotonin, a feel good hormone that among other things contributes to a sense of well being. After sunset, the body halts the production of serotonin and releases melatonin, the sleep hormone. Both the hormones are vital for mental and physical health. Most importantly, it determines when your body is primed for being awake or asleep. However, the circadian rhythm needs signals from the external environment—most importantly daylight and darkness—to adjust itself. Blue-wavelength light stimulates sensors in your eyes to send signals to your brain's internal clock. Getting blue light, especially from the sun, in the daytime helps you stay alert while improving performance and mood.

The sun is a natural source of radiant energy. The sunlight is much richer in shorter wavelength blue light than any other artificial light sources. Studies have suggested that time spent outdoors in sunlight is protective against occurrence and development of myopia. It has been shown that time spent in sunlight can help control the eye elongation that can affect refractive development and reverse myopia. In addition the research also shows that blue light is vital for reduction in astigmatism during development.

There are bad effects also. The immediate effect of prolong exposure to blue light leads to glare, eye strain, headache, fatigue, and insomnia. Studies have also shown that the constant exposure to blue light over time can damage retinal cells and cause vision problems such as age-related macular degeneration. It can also contribute to cataracts, eye cancer and growths on the clear covering over the white part of the eye. Dry eyes are another problem that may occur due to over exposure to blue light. The microvilli on the epithelial layer of the corneal epithelium lose the support and stability of the tear film, leading to formation of dry eyes. According to a vision study by the National Eye Institute, children are more at risk than adults because their eyes absorb more blue light from digital devices.

It is, therefore, incorrect to say that all blue light from 380 nm to 510 nm are bad for eyes and overall well being of the people. The researchers have divided the blue light into two categories as shown in **Figure 10.5**.

- High energy visible blue (HEV)
- Low energy visible blue (LEV).

LEV Blue lies above 435 nm and it gives the perception of blue - turquoise light. We need LEV Blue for our well being. HEV lies below

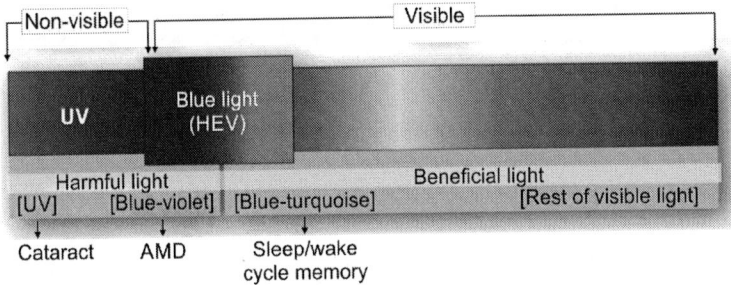

Fig. 10.5: Two types of blue light.

435 nm and it gives the perception of blue- violet light. HEV blue light are harmful and therefore needs to be prevented to transmit through the eyes structure.

Exposure to blue light during daytime hours helps maintain a healthful circadian rhythm. Too much exposure to blue light late at night through digital devices can disturb the wake and sleep cycle, leading to problems sleeping and daytime tiredness. Therefore, it is good that we should minimize the exposure of eyes to blue light during the night time to avoid the effect of blue light on the secretion of melatonin, so as to ensure good sleep and eye closure time. Blue light in the night tricks the brain into thinking that it's daytime, which inhibits the production of melatonin and reduces both the quantity and quality of your sleep.

Recently there has been a lot of buzz around Blue Cut lenses which are designed to minimize the transmission blue light to eyes. Blue cut lenses may feature layered substrates or blue light blocking coatings. Some blue-light-blocking lenses are infused with melanin, which is naturally found in the skin. They may have a brownish-yellow tint. This helps filtering out blue light. The use of blue cut lenses may be useful in the night while working on digital devices. It may help to normalize the circadian rhythm and minimize the risk of macular degeneration at the later part of the life. The capacity of blue light prevention can differ from 10% to 90%, depending upon the quality of the blue cut filter. A good quality blue cut lenses prevents the transmission of high energy visible blue and allows the transmission of low energy visible blue light.

Multiple Choice Questions-Answers

1. Which of the following is the symptom of light sensitivity?
   a. Rapid blinking and poor concentration
   b. Narrowing of the palpebral aperture
   c. Dark adaptation
   d. All of the above

2. Which of the following is not considered to be the effect of glare?
   a. Reduced contrast sensitivity
   b. Reduced color discrimination
   c. Reduced visual field
   d. Poor dark adaptation

3. Which of the following does not form the part of the sequential management consideration for glare for a subject who presents the symptoms of computer vision syndrome (CVS)?
   a. Room light illumination
   b. The screen brightness adjustment
   c. Reorientation of workstation
   d. Prescribe added lenses

Answer Key

| 1. | (d) | 2. | (c) | 3. | (d) |

Self-Practice Questions

1. What may cause glare for visual display unit (VDU) user? Will anti-reflective coating on eyeglasses eliminate the effect of glare?
2. How would you diagnose the glare problem for a patient who has come to you with complaints of computer-related vision problem? What remedial measures would you suggest?
3. Differentiate between Glare and Reflection. How do they affect people working on VDUs?

CHAPTER 11

Presbyopia and Computer Use

SYMPTOMS

The blurred near vision signals the onset of presbyopia. A presbyopic patient shows the following symptoms in common:
- Delay in focusing at near
- Ocular discomfort
- Headache
- Asthenopia
- Fatigue with reading
- Drowsiness while prolonged near work
- Increased near-working distance
- Need for brighter light for reading
- Pulling sensation or eyestrain while reading.

RATIONALE

Presbyopia is an age-related visual impairment. It results from the gradual decrease in amplitude of accommodation expected with age and can have multiple effects on quality of vision and quality of life. As the amplitude of accommodation diminishes, the range of clear vision may become inadequate for the patient's commonly performed near and extended near-vision tasks. The need for amplitude of accommodation is more at near distance than at extended near distance. The bottom line is that presbyopia is not just the problem of near vision at 40 cm; it is a problem of reduced vision at various reading distances. The patient who is working on a computer also notices blur vision at the computer monitor which is usually kept at 50–70 cm. The blurring at this distance is comparatively less as accommodative demand at this distance is comparatively less. Those who are involved more in near-vision tasks are likely to have more difficulty. Because the need to read and work at near and intermediate distances is important in all industrialized societies, presbyopia has both clinical and social significance. The patient complains that his hands are shorter to enable them to read. If the condition remains untreated, it causes significant functional visual disability. The condition is irreversible and is an evolutionary blunder that comes as a psychological shock **(Fig. 11.1)**.

DIAGNOSIS OF PRESBYOPIA

Presbyopia can be diagnosed by following clinical care are shown in **Flowchart 11.1**.

Patient History

The patient history is probably the most important tool to diagnose the onset of presbyopia. The patient may complain in different ways. An example may be, "My arms are not long enough." Others may complain of problem in threading a needle. A patient who wears minus spectacles may report that removing the spectacles for near-vision task helps him to read. The medical history is equally important, especially in the diagnosis of premature presbyopia, particularly when the

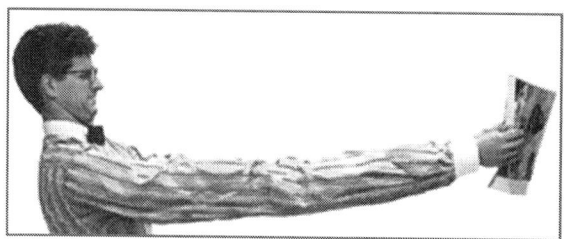

Fig. 11.1: Presbyopic patient.
(*Courtesy:* Essilor India Pvt Ltd)

Flowchart 11.1: Diagnosing presbyopia.

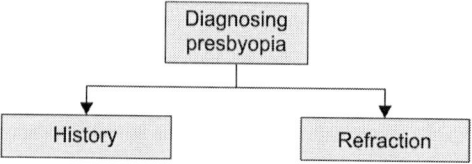

patient has significant systemic disease. Conditions such as diabetes mellitus, vascular disease, neurological disorders, trauma, or the use of certain medications may contribute to premature presbyopia. Premature presbyopia suggests an associated condition that needs attention. Obtaining information about vocational and avocational activities is important in the diagnosis of presbyopia.

Refraction

A careful distance refraction provides the foundation for determining the management of presbyopia. The optical correction for presbyopia is the sum of the refractive correction for distance correction plus the power of the near addition. An alternative way to deal with presbyopia is called monovision. In monovision, a patient's dominant eye is given a distance prescription, while the other eye is given a near prescription. Contact lens practitioners and refractive surgeons practice monovision very often to treat their presbyopic patients. While monovision can decrease the need for reading glasses, it can take some time to get used to. Monovision can affect depth perception, and you may not feel comfortable driving or reading for extended periods.

Determine the Near Addition

The presbyopia is corrected with near addition or "add." The "add" is the additional plus lens prescribed over the distance correction. The strength of the near add depends upon the age, the preferred working distance, and the best corrected distance visual acuity as shown in **Flowchart 11.2**.

The strength of near "add" increases as the age increases. The goal is to find lowest plus that gives clearest vision at required near

Flowchart 11.2: Three factors that dictate the strength of add.

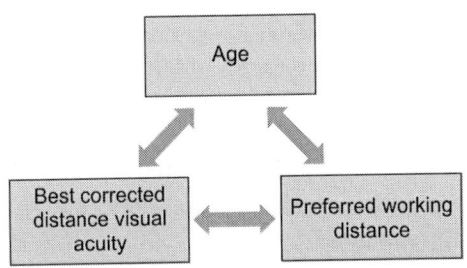

Flowchart 11.3: Tests for near addition.

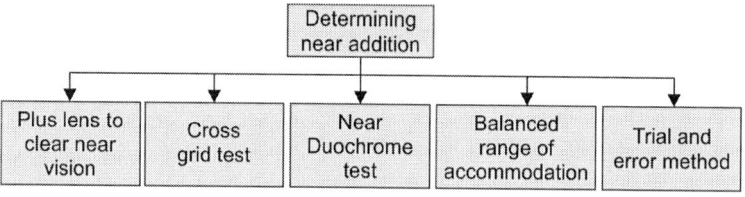

distance. Usually, near add should be verified with both eyes together and the near acuity should be equivalent to that of the distance. If not, you may consider increasing the near add. Ideally, the near add for both eyes should be the same. However, near add should always be responsive to the patient's visual needs. The final consideration is the patient's comfort and his satisfaction. Different methods may be applied to perform the test for near addition. The most common of them are shown in **Flowchart 11.3**.

Plus Lens to Clear Near Vision

This is the most common method to determine the required near addition. Plus power over the distance correction is increased until clear near vision is achieved. The test may be performed monocularly or binocularly. The binocular procedure yields a lower addition power due to convergent accommodation. While performing this test, the clinician should take care to ensure a patient's habitual viewing circumstances, such as working distance and lighting.

Cross Grid Test (Fig. 11.2)

- Use phoropter.
- Place the cross grid at a near point distance.
- Reduce room illumination.
- Put + and – 0.50 D cross cylinder with minus axis vertically in front of both eyes with distance correction in place.
- Now ask the patient which set of lines are clear and sharper—horizontal or vertical.
- Expected answer: Horizontal lines
- Add plus lens binocularly until vertical lines are clear and sharper.
- Then reduce plus to achieve equal clarity and sharpness.
- That is the end point.

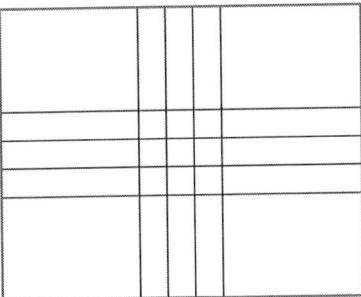

Fig. 11.2: Cross grid test.

Near Duochrome Test

- Ask the patient to hold the Near Duochrome Test in his hand with distance correction in place in the trial frame at a distance as decided.
- A Duochrome test with black rings or letters may be used. Ask the patient to keep both eyes open and look at the black rings, if a black ring is used. Ask him to identify which black ring is clearer or darker—one on the red background or one on the green background. Three possible responses can be expected:
  - Either a black ring on a green background is clearer and darker which indicates the need for plus lens or
  - A black ring on the red background is clearer and darker which indicates the need for reduction of plus power.
  - Rings on both sides—red and green background—appear similar.

Uncorrected or undercorrected presbyopes will have marked green preference. In a young patient with active accommodation, the preference for red and green will alternate indicating that there is no need for any near "add." The most important thing to note is that this test applies only for a particular fixation distance used during the test. If the test distance is moved toward the eyes, the green preference will be dominant and if the test distance is taken away from the fixation point, the red preference will become dominant.

Balanced Range of Accommodation

NRA determines the maximum ability to relax accommodation while maintaining single and clear binocular vision at reading distance. PRA determines the maximum ability to accommodate while maintaining single and clear, single binocular vision at reading distance. NRA is determined by adding plus power lens binocularly until the patient is no longer able to read the fine prints on the test card. The PRA is determined by adding minus power lenses until the patient is no longer able to read the fine prints. The difference between the NRA and the PRA is called the relative accommodative amplitude. Using these data, the clinician may achieve the indicated addition as under:

Example: PRA – 0.50 D
NRA + 2.00 D
Range 2.50

Therefore, the indicated required addition is + 2.00 – (2.50/2) = +0.75 D.

Trial and Error Method

Near addition may be prescribed by the trial-and-error method. In this process, near addition is decided based on the age of the patient and the lenses are put in the trial frame to verify that vision is fairly good and the patient is comfortable at his usual working distance. One problem with this approach is that it assumes that all individuals of the same age have the same amplitude of accommodation, which is not the case in practice. The typical age with correspondingly required near addition may be designed as given in **Table 11.1**.

Once the near addition is determined as above, put the proposed near addition in the trial frame with distance correction and confirm that vision is fairly good and the patient is comfortable at his usual working distance.

Table 11.1: Typical age with correspondingly required near addition.

Age	Near addition
40 years	0.75 D
42 years	1.00 D
44 years	1.50 D
46 years	1.75 D
48 years	2.00 D
50 years	2.25 D

COMPUTER AND PRESBYOPIA

When the computers first appeared on the working desks, a new uncovered issue related to presbyopia was unleashed. A good number of research papers were published about the ergonomics of the computer workstation and visual demands of the computers. Conferences were held, and books and articles were published. The reasons were fairly simple—the traditional presbyopic correction at 40 cm was not good enough to provide the comfortable vision at the computer screen. Researchers discovered that there was considerable change in the viewing distance and viewing angle while working on the computers than the most common correction designed to provide at 40 cm with a downward gaze angle of 25-30°. The normal glasses that meet their visual needs for most other tasks usually do not properly correct their vision for computer display. The computer display is usually farther away at around 50-70 cm than the usual reading distance. Also, the computer display is higher which demands the patient to have downward gaze of only 10-20°. A presbyope who tries to wear his usual multifocal correction at the computer either does not see the computer display clearly or needs to assume an awkward posture, resulting in neck and back strain. Most commonly, a presbyope needs to inch closer to the screen and tilt his head backward; the former is bad for the back and the latter is bad for the neck. This is true for bifocal lenses and even for progressive addition lenses. Although progressive addition lenses provide a region with an intermediate addition, this is the portion of the lens with the narrowest field of clear vision. The person wearing progressive addition lens must continuously try and find the small sweet spot on the lens and use his neck to move the head rather than moving the eyes. Nearly all computer users have some viewing requirements at 40 cm. Distance visual needs are often considerably less important for them when they are on the computer and it is, therefore, often compromised in the interests of best meeting the intermediate and near tasks. Today, computers are accepted as an integral part of life and are considered as traits of advancement in trade, industry, and business; there will not be any surprise that most people will experience these visual problems some time or the other. It is, therefore, the responsibility of the eye care practitioners to consider these aspects while examining the patient and prescribing him with suitable correction.

TREATING PRESBYOPIC PATIENTS FOR COMPUTER WORK WITH LENSES

The clinical care to treat presbyopic patients for computer display is to be achieved in two steps as shown in **Figure 11.3**.

The determination of addition required for a presbyope computer user has to be ideally determined in two separate steps. The first step is to determine the correct near addition at a usual near working distance of 40 cm. Once this is done, the enhancement has to be made to achieve at the correct addition required for computer display. In order to determine the correct addition required for computer display, it is useful to know how far the computer display is from the eyes and also how far the other near work is from the patient's eyes. Care must be ensured to obtain the information as patients are not very good at providing this information without making a direct measurement. Another important factor to be considered before determining addition for computer display is to know patient's computer workstation arrangement as there is always a possibility that the current working station arrangement may be found to be faulty. In such a case, it is important to counsel the patient to reorganize the working station arrangement, and accordingly the addition for computer display is determined. Some patients who are fighting the onset of presbyopia have learnt to push their computer screen away from them. Once the correct computer screen location is determined, the prescription should be designed at the designated location. However, final prescription determination is often best determined by demonstration. It may be very effective to make the

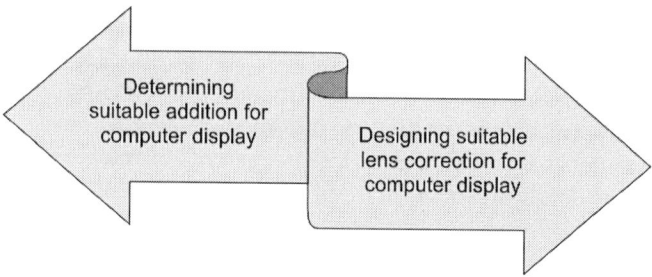

Fig. 11.3: Two step method for determining and designing the near correction for presbyopic computer user.

final prescription measurements in free space by seating the patient at a computer screen. A simulated computer screen, including the PRIO unit, is available to serve the purpose. This also reminds the patient about the special care he is receiving for his computer work. The patient intermediate distance correction, near vision correction, and distance vision correction should be separately determined and a prescription and lens design prescribed accordingly. Many a times, distance visual need is compromised in the interest of best meeting the intermediate and near needs.

Once the correction for computer display is determined, the suitable lenses may be prescribed. There are several spectacle options available. Out of necessity, most of them acquire a lens correction that suits their needs and lifestyle. An improper lens design may cause compromised visual performance, eye-related symptoms, and awkward posture with ensuing musculoskeletal symptoms, thereby reducing the work efficiency and ultimately early retirement. Properly designed work-related glasses provide better vision and comfort during the work. These specialty glasses called "task-specific" or "occupational glasses" are designed to meet the visual needs of the occupation only.

The fundamental visual limitation in the spectacle correction of presbyopia is that because presbyopia results in a fixed focus eye, a refractive correction can only correct a single viewing distance, although in reality there is a range of clear vision. This problem is resolved to some extent by wearing multifocal lenses in which the power of the lens varies depending on the gaze angle. Because distance objects are generally higher in the field of view and near objects lower, optical correction of presbyopia generally provides the distance correction in the top of the lens and near correction in the bottom of the lens. The power in the bottom of the lens is usually that will provide clear vision at 40 cm. This is a typical reading distance and a standard near testing distance used by eye doctors. If the viewing distance and/or gaze requirements of the job are different than this, then different glasses are indicated for the job. This is particularly true for the patients who perform their visual task at intermediate viewing distance (50–70 cm) and/or for those with needs to see at near or intermediate viewing distance straight ahead or overhead.

Flowchart 11.4: Lens options for presbyope computer user.

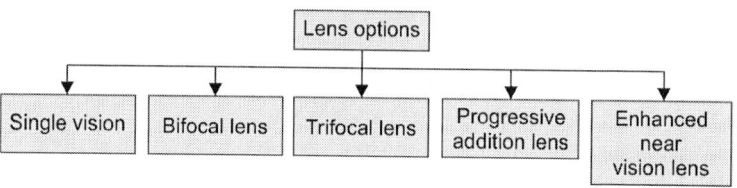

Some workstations enable the worker to assume a reclined position. This is common for people who spend many continuous hours at a workstation. If they recline, it results in the computer screen being higher than the eyes. When prescribing for these people, the backward head tilt needs to be considered in the design of any multifocal lens. The nature and style of work process is also an important factor. For example, patients engaged in data entry need to move their eyes a lot between the source document and the computer display. The others may be operating with a very large screen with large images or text or without a requirement to see small detail. In such cases, it may be advantageous to work with a little longer distance. The avid use of computer and occasional use of computer also make a difference. The various lens options that may be prescribed are shown in **Flowchart 11.4**.

Single-Vision Lenses

A single-vision correction offers the advantage of a large, clear field of vision, and it is also the least expensive option. This may be the option of choice for the new emergent presbyope who still has enough remaining accommodation to see clearly at 40 cm with the addition for the computer distance. If it is possible to accomplish without compromising the patient's near vision, trim the addition on the lower side to decrease the distance blur. The distance blur through this single-vision prescription should be demonstrated to the patient. However, if the distant blur is disturbing to the patient, another design is indicated. Moderate-to-high myopes usually prefer single-vision correction trimmed for working distance.

Bifocal Lenses

An advanced presbyope may be more comfortable with flat top bifocal. In such a case, the top portion of the lens contains the intermediate

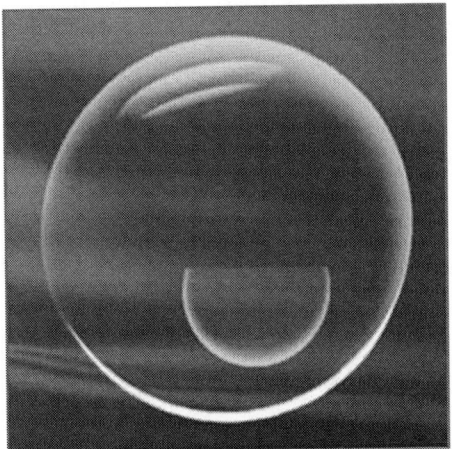

Fig. 11.4: Bifocal lenses.

prescription and the bottom segment contains the near prescription for 40 cm. The distance blur through the top portion of the lens is demonstrated to the patient. The intermediate power may be trimmed a bit to lessen the distance blur. The prescription should be written with a note that it is for computer use only. In nearly all such cases, the bifocal needs to be fitted a little higher than normal and the patient needs to be aware that the bifocal location makes it difficult to walk around the office and the lens is not useful for meeting normal distance visual requirements **(Fig. 11.4)**.

Trifocal Lenses

Trifocal lenses can be good for more advanced presbyopes who are intolerant to distant blur and require clear vision at their computer distance. These patients use bifocals or trifocals for their general wear and are averse to progressives. Hence, occupational enhanced near-vision lens is also inappropriate for them **(Fig. 11.5)**.

Progressive Addition Lenses

Progressive addition lenses are another common lens design used to correct presbyopia. These lenses are characterized by a smooth continuous change of power across the lens surface, but with undesired aberrations at the lower periphery on either side. The

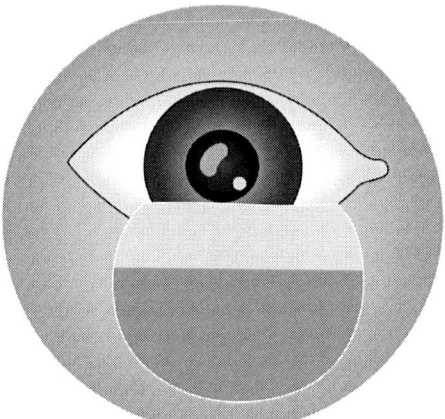

Fig. 11.5: Trifocal lens.

smooth change in the power across the lens surface provides the user a region with intermediate power. It is for this reason that they are most commonly prescribed for computer use. It is, therefore, important to understand that the region for intermediate power is a very narrow field of clear vision. If the patient requires significant viewing at an intermediate distance or spend most of his day on a computer, he must continuously find the sweet spot in the lens and use his neck to move the head rather than his eyes. This may cause musculoskeletal stress and may reduce the field of view. However, progressive addition lenses are a good arrangement for distance vision, near vision, and intermediate distance vision in one single spectacle and are really very effective for an intermittent short-term computer user. In such a situation, the work period is shorter and the neck movement can be tolerated for a short period **(Figs. 11.6A and B)**.

Occupational Enhanced Near-Vision Lenses

Occupational enhanced near-vision lenses are specially designed lenses that meet the presbyopic demands of the patients with extensive intermediate viewing needs, such as computer users, assembly line workers, clerks, and general office work. The lens design provides a reasonably large intermediate vision on the top of the lens to enable them to navigate the workplace. The magnitude of unwanted aberrations in occupational enhanced near-vision lenses is

Chapter 11: Presbyopia and Computer Use

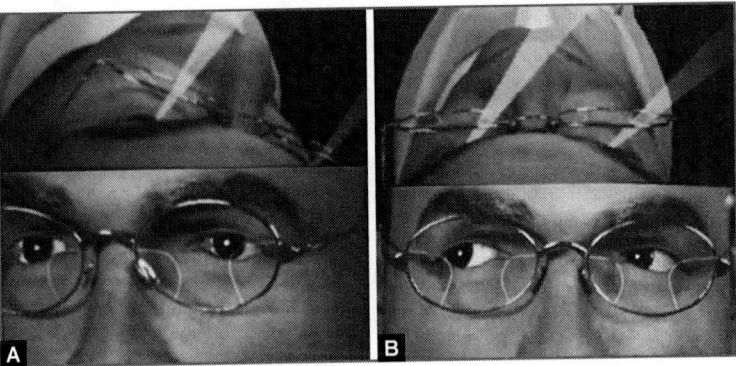

Figs. 11.6A and B: Progressive addition lens (PALs): (A) Head movement is essential for correct use of PALs for lateral gazing; (B) Only eye movement is incorrect way of using PALs.

significantly less than that in a progressive addition lens because the total power change is less, resulting in wider viewing zones compared to the progressive addition lens. However, they do not meet general viewing needs outside of the workplace.

Occupational enhanced near-vision lenses can be very successful in meeting the visual demands of most presbyopic computer users. A favorable consideration is that the patient is using progressive addition lenses for general use and occupational enhanced near-vision lenses for computer use. Patients must be counseled that these lenses are specially designed for use at the computer and that they should not be worn for other tasks, especially driving.

There is no one specific solution as computer glasses that fits all or is the best for everybody. Visual ability and personal preferences of a computer operator, the type of work, the distance between the computer user's eyes and the monitor, and lighting design in any given workplace are factors that should be taken into consideration while selecting computer glasses. Each of the options listed above can be beneficial for computer users, if properly fitted and recorrected as needed. However, it is very important that the selection of computer glasses is made based on consultation with an eye specialist who is knowledgeable in problems specific to the regular use of a computer. But the fact remains that counseling is the most important aspect that they require a separate pair of spectacle for their computer use.

Multiple Choice Questions-Answers

1. **Near addition should be prescribed....**
   a. Based upon a patient's age
   b. Based upon a monocular test of near addition
   c. Based upon subjective examination and patient's visual needs
   d. All of the above

2. **The onset of presbyopia does not depend on which of the following?**
   a. Near-vision task
   b. Sex of the patients
   c. Refractive state of the patients
   d. Amplitude of accommodation

3. **Mr Raman, aged 44, is working in a software company. He has data-feeding job from hardcopy. His current prescription shows that he is hyperopic with +1.00 Dsph +0.75 Dcyl × 180 in both eyes with a near addition of +1.50 Dsph. Which of the following solutions would help him to enhance the visual performance and minimize the disadvantage to improve occupational performance?**
   a. Regressive lens
   b. Progressive lens
   c. Aggressive lens
   d. Suppressive lens

Answer Key

| 1. | (c) | 2. | (b) | 3. | (a) |

Self-Practice Questions

1. Explain how symptoms of presbyopic patients would be related to the design of the prescription used for computer use.
2. A 45-year-old with a moderate amount of hypermetropia using progressive addition lenses for his all-day activities finds that he is having difficulty in feeding data in computer from source documents. What might you recommend?
3. A new bifocal wearer reports that his bifocal lenses are working very well for most of his daily life activities. However, he found that his vision is not clear in two situations: Viewing the visual display unit (VDU) screen while sitting on his office desk and while reading books lying in bed at night. What is the most likely cause of these difficulties? What are possible solutions?

CHAPTER 12

Computer-workstation Arrangement

Law 3 of Laws of Computer Vision says that visual abilities determine visual postures which will also be influenced by visual environment. This is based on the assumption that human eyes take the lead in deciding the bodily posture. Nature has designed our visual system to be so dominant that we alter our bodily posture to accommodate any deficiency in the way we see. If the task is visually demanding, the body locates the eyes at a position where they can perform the visual task comfortably but assumes an awkward posture that results in musculoskeletal problems. Unhygienic visual environment adds to it.

The straightforward meaning is that we need to be aware of how the design and the arrangement of the equipment in our computer workstation can affect our comfort, health, and productivity. This is very important to minimize the work-related musculoskeletal difficulties, such as carpal tunnel syndrome, back pain, and neck pain that are commonly seen with computer workers. Another important issue that needs to be kept in mind while designing furniture and fixture is the fact that the human body is designed for movement. The position that does not allow any body movement while working leads to more fatigue than the position that allows moderate movement. When the body is still, circulation is slowed and as a result fewer nutrients are delivered to the muscles. The result can be musculoskeletal discomfort and pain.

Now, the question arises: why it is important for an optometrist to have an idea about computer workstation designs? Yes, it may not be very important for an optometrist to know about it if he is in general practice. But this is very important for an optometrist who specializes in the practice of computer vision syndrome. The reasons

Flowchart 12.1: Factors affecting computer workstation.

```
                    Body
                 posture of
                  computer
                    user
                      |
  Furniture  ——  Factors    ——  Computer
    and          affecting       hardware and
   fixture       computer        attachment
                 workstation     arrange-
                                 ment
                      |
                  Computer
                   display
```

are simple. Knowing information about a computer workstation forms an important part of history taking that allows him to relate the signs and symptoms to actual cause. In turn, it helps him to design a comprehensive treatment plan for the patient. The various workstation-related factors that are important for him are shown in the **Flowchart 12.1**.

ISSUES RELATED TO BODY POSTURE

A neutral body posture lets you work with comfort and ease for which it is essential that the workstation is matched to the worker. A mismatch workstation may force uncomfortable posture that leads the symptoms of CVS. Several factors are important to ensure neutral body posture while working on a computer. The important among them are shown in **Flowchart 12.2**.

- A down-ocular gaze angle of 15–20° relative to straight-ahead gaze is more ideal for optimal performance as the effect on near-triad function is relatively insignificant. When we look down, our eyes converge, accommodate to focus, and pupils constrict that alter the depth of focus. The condition is just opposite when we look

Chapter 12: Computer-workstation Arrangement

Flowchart 12.2: Body posture issues.

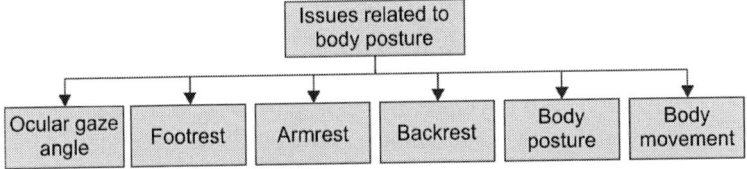

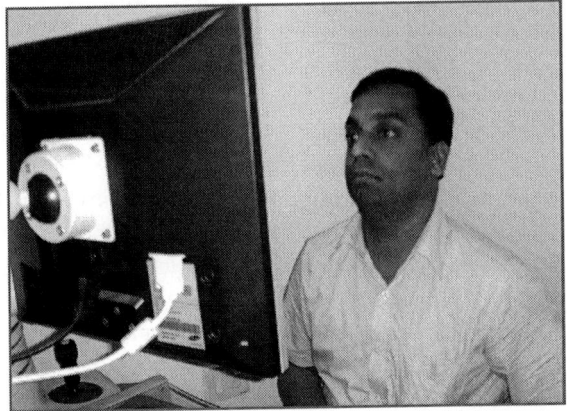

Fig. 12.1: Display screen at a higher position, not a correct position.

straight ahead or upward. In such a position, it is harder to focus for close objects. There are some accommodative advantages to having down-ocular gaze in the form of accommodative convergence which is mainly a reflex convergence. This is also supported when we study the optical corrections available for presbyopia. All the bifocal and multifocal lenses have near-viewing zones located in the lower portion so that the near-viewing angle is 20–25° below the horizontal line of sight. This location has been empirically determined to be comfortable for the presbyopic patients **(Fig. 12.1)**.

- Resting of feet on the floor while working on computers for a long period of time allows support for legs that reduces pressure on the lower back and prevents leg swelling. In case the height of the chair does not allow for the same, a separate footrest may be used.
- It is also important to have support for the forearm while working with a mouse or keyboard in order to reduce tension, mainly in

the neck and shoulder muscles as well as localized pressure on the wrist. Together with the arm rest, a soft wrist rest in front of keyboard or mouse is helpful to prevent carpal tunnel syndrome.
- While sitting vertically straight on a chair, our back has to be fully supported with backrest. This is important to reduce stress and strain on the muscles, tendons, and skeletal system and to reduce the risk of developing a musculoskeletal problem.
- Body posture as a whole is very important while seating for a longer duration of time in one position. Having just one part of our body out of neutral posture can affect the rest of the posture. It is, therefore, essential that a comfortable working posture in which all our joints are naturally aligned has to be maintained to reduce the musculoskeletal disorder.
- Regardless of how good our posture may be, sitting still for a long period of time is not healthy. Small changes in the posture at about every 15 minutes flex the body muscles. Larger changes in posture are also important. It may be a good idea to stand up, stretch, or walk around for 1 or 2 minutes at a regular interval.

ISSUES RELATED TO FURNITURE AND FIXTURE

The designing and arrangement of furniture and fixture influence the visual comfort, visual efficiency, and body posture. The following factors are important as far as issues related to furniture and fixtures are concerned **(Flowchart 12.3)**.
- The distance between the eyes and the computer monitor determines the working viewing distance. There are several factors to be considered while deciding onto the viewing distance. Most researchers support the longer viewing distance because of the least visual demand on the visual system. But this is limited by availability of space and operational ease. It may also put stress

Flowchart 12.3: Computer station: Furniture and fixture.

```
                    Issues related to
                furniture and fixture
    ┌──────────┬──────────┬──────┬──────────┬──────────┐
  Viewing    Viewing    Chair   Computer   Lighting
  distance   height             desk
```

on torso because of forward leaning. At a closer distance, our eyes are at a constant accommodative state that results in early fatigue and other symptoms. Some researchers are of the opinion that the greatest visual comfort is achieved when working at resting point of accommodation or resting point of vergence. However, they vary with different persons and also with age. This may not be possible because of availability of space in the office. The most commonly accepted distance where the computer display should be placed is 50–70 cm from eyes. However, screen size and font size used while working should be taken into consideration while deciding onto it.

- The height of a computer monitor determines the working viewing height. Several factors influence this decision. The objects lying at distance are generally placed higher in the field of view and the objects lying at the near distance are placed lower. This is well accepted by the ophthalmic lens designers when they designed all the optical correction for the presbyopia providing distance correction at the top of the lens and near correction at the bottom of the lens. But since the advent of computers in the close work, the viewing height has become an important issue as it exposes the user to a different ergonomic world. The optimal height of the screen depends on several factors, and people also adapt to the vertical location of their task by changing their gaze angle or by changing neck position or both. If the computer display is kept higher, it forces the user to keep his eyes wide open and exposes him to more discomfort glare. A higher gaze angle results in a greater exposed ocular surface, resulting in an increased amount of tear evaporation and adding to dry eye problem. There are some accommodative advantages to having down gaze as against straight-ahead gaze. It has been studied that the amplitude of accommodation is greater with downward-viewing position compared to upward-viewing position. Also, while looking down, your eyes have a natural tendency to turn inward and focus for near objects. The opposite is true for looking straight ahead or upward—your eyes tend to turn outward and focus at a distance, and you will have to work harder to focus for close objects with your head in this position. All these indicate better performance and comfort with down gaze compared to up gaze. It justifies

keeping the computer display slightly below the horizontal visual line of the user so that the user has a down-gaze angle of 15–20° relative to straight-ahead gaze.
- A comfortable chair is most important for the computer user as he spends almost the entire day sitting on it. It must be designed as per his body with easily adjustable and reachable controls. The chair should have five legs with lockable casters to prevent tipping and allow easy roll on the floor. It should have large, wide, and soft-padded two armrests to support the forearm. The backrest should be large enough to support the entire back and should contour to the curve of the lower back.
- The computer desk should provide adequate space to place both the feet together with footrest if needed. The top of the desk should be laminated with a matte surface to minimize the glare. It should be large enough to accommodate all the parts of the computer system with all attachments needed to work efficiently. It should also have two accessory drawers, pullout keyboard tray with safety stop, and elevated shelf to accommodate the printer.
- Good lighting is very critical for a computer working station. Good lighting is the situation when all the visual objects in the field of view are uniformly or near uniformly illuminated. Working on computers is different than working with paper and writing materials. Computers are self-illuminated, whereas papers need illumination from different sources. This is one of the reasons for discomfort glare. The other glare sources are bright open windows, horizontal fixation point, white paper on desk, any glossy surface in the field of view, white tabletops, and shiny finish walls. There are basically two types of lighting arrangements—overall lighting and task-specific lighting. Task-specific lighting can put light directly on the specific object in such a way that it illuminates the object of interest uniformly and adequately and does not hit the eyes directly. While installing overall lighting, care should be taken to ensure at least 300–500 lux. There are different types of lights available. Some of the examples are fluorescent lamps, tungsten halogen lamps, incandescent lamps, and mercury and metal-halide lamps. Tubular fluorescent lamps are one of the most common sources of commercial lighting and are also among the most efficient. Light fittings should be installed in such a way so

as to ensure uniform light distribution to prevent discomfort glare. In a large office where a series of overhead lights are installed, it is always better if the workers look along the rows of lights while viewing a computer display rather than across the rows.

ISSUES RELATED TO HARDWARE AND ATTACHMENT

The issues related to hardware and attachment are shown in **Flowchart 12.4**.

Computer Monitor

A correct placement of monitor is very important to minimize the symptoms of computer vision syndrome. The following issues need to be addressed:

- **Monitor distance:** Place the monitor at a distance of 50–70 cm from the eyes. If you are presbyopic, set the distance to your refractive correction.
- **Monitor height:** Adjust the height of the monitor screen to allow gazing slightly down to view the center of the screen.
- **Monitor angle:** Tilt the monitor screen slightly to accommodate your line of sight. If you are using bifocal glasses, monitor position might be shifted lower.
- **Monitor size:** Monitor should be large enough to display a sizeable amount of information.

Keyboard

Placement of keyboard determines the comfort for forearm, wrist, and shoulder. The most comfortable position for the wrist is straight and extended 10–20° upward. A soft-padded wrist rest in front of the keyboard is helpful. The height of the keyboard depends on the height

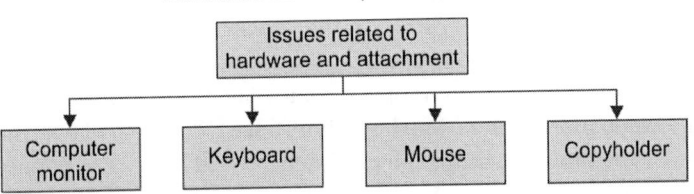

Flowchart 12.4: Computer accessories.

of the work surface and chair. To reduce tension in your shoulder muscles, the keyboard should be low enough so that your arms are relaxed at your sides.

Mouse

The mouse should be located immediately next to the keyboard so that reaching is easy. Placing mouse too far away, or too low, or too much on one side can cause shoulder, wrist, elbow, and forearm discomfort.

Copyholder

A document holder should be stable, but you should be able to adjust its height, position, distance, and angle of view. Keep the ocular dominancy in your mind while deciding to place monitor screen and the copyholder. If you need to copy from the source document, place the source document towards your dominant eye next to your computer monitor. This will allow you to look from the screen to document holder with little ease and less movement of neck.

ISSUES RELATED TO COMPUTER DISPLAY

Human performance and comfort are related to the legibility, readability, or both of the computer display. Improving the legibility of the display is one of the simplest ways to improve the visual environment for a computer user. The CVS specialist optometrist is supposed to educate the computer user on the effect of poor computer display quality on their visual performance and give him necessary guidance on how to maximize the display images. The following factors with respect to computer display influence the legibility and readability or both of the display (**Flowchart 12.5**).

Resolution

For computer displays, the resolution of an image refers to the optical quality and density of pixels on the screen and to the total number of pixels displayed on the screen. The most common representation of the resolution of computer monitor is dot pitch or the distance between pixel centers. Most monitors have a dot pitch of 0.28 mm or less. The dot pitch limits the pixel density and hence the fineness of details. Smaller values are desirable.

Flowchart 12.5: Computer display determinants.

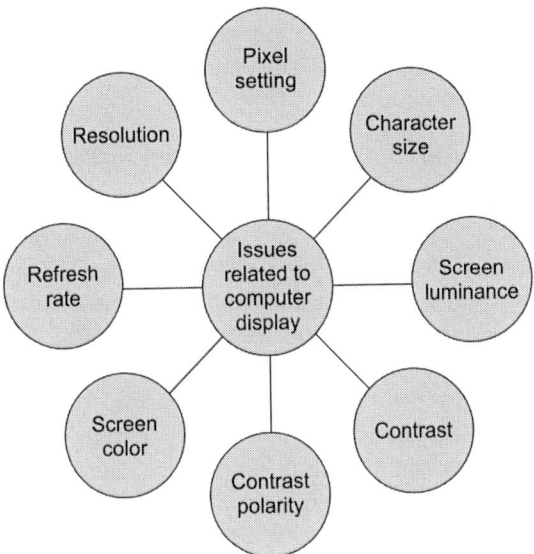

Pixel Settings

Pixel settings represent the maximum number of pixels that can be displayed. The control panel provides the option to adjust the display settings. Higher pixel settings allow more documents or windows to be seen simultaneously on the screen. The user should select the settings that work best for him.

Character Size

The size of character on the display is important for the efficient function and comfort. The character size should be large than threshold near acuity, keeping in mind the image compromise inherent to computer display.

Screen Luminance

Monitors with the capability of displaying high screen luminance are usually desirable. Small improvements in vision have been shown with increased luminance. However, the display luminance is to be balanced with other visual targets.

Contrast

High contrast makes character more legible on the display. Typically, the contrast is better with LCD display than with CRT as it minimizes the screen reflection.

Contrast Polarity

It is always better to use dark characters on a light background. With a white background screen, the brightness of the screen is a better match for the surrounding room. Also, a dark background screen is more prone to reflection problem. The reflections result in the entire background becoming brighter, therefore decreasing the contrast of the light characters on the dark background. With white background screens, it is possible to operate more comfortably in an office with normal light illumination. With dark background screens, it is necessary to reduce the lighting in the office. Moreover, black letters on a white background are the normally same as those of paper task.

Screen Color

The color presented on a computer display is limited by the capability of the display and the graphic card. Most computers allow changing the color settings from the control panel.

Refresh Rate

It is the speed at which the screen is repainted. The higher the refresh rate, the steadier will be the screen image.

IDEAL SITTING POSTURE WHILE WORKING ON A COMPUTER

- Head slightly tilted downward.
- Shoulders relaxed, not elevated, hunched, or rotated forward.
- Elbow close to your sides and bent at about 90° angle.
- Use the chair's backrest to support your lower back or lumbar curve.
- Sit with your entire body upright or leaning slightly back.
- Keep your wrists straight while you work, not bent up, down, or to the sides.
- Place your feet slightly out in front of your knees and make sure that they are comfortably supported, either by the floor or by a footrest (**Fig. 12.2**).

Chapter 12: Computer-workstation Arrangement

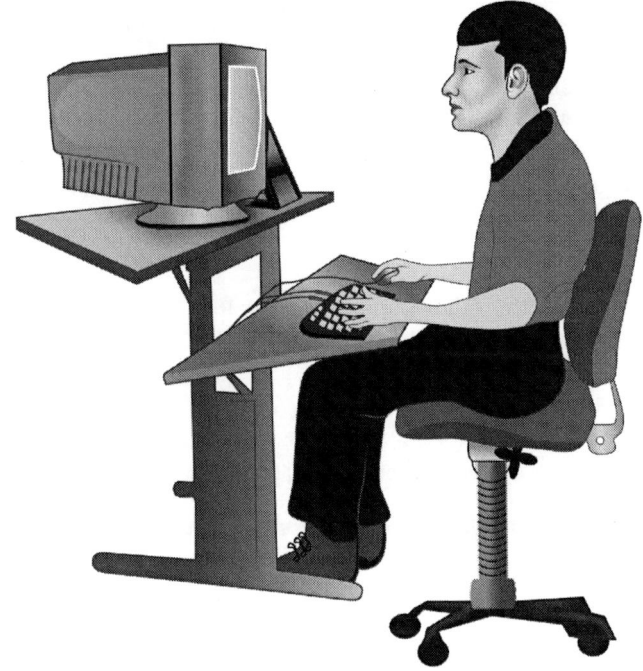

Fig. 12.2: Comfortable sitting posture.

IDEAL COMPUTER WORKSTATION

- Work area should be large enough to provide some body movements in addition to be enough for equipment and other accessories.
- Place those items in your nearest reach which are used more frequently.
- Avoid overcrowding.
- Do not direct the warm airflow from CPU toward you.
- Monitor should be placed at a correct distance and height.
- Copyholder and other accessories are at an appropriate position.
- Adequate overall lighting should be arranged, as explained earlier.
- Provision for task-specific light.
- Comfortable chair.
- Large-sized monitor with good pixel setting.

Chapter 12: Computer Workstation Arrangement

Multiple Choice Questions-Answers

1. Which of the following may happen because of the improper placement of the keyboard?
   a. Tendonitis of wrist
   b. Back pain
   c. Migraine headache
   d. Stress fracture

2. Which of the following is not a healthy habit to follow while working on visual display units (VDUs)?
   a. Keyboard should be placed on a shelf below the desktop
   b. Seat should not cause pressure on the knees
   c. Seat should support the lower back
   d. Feet should be allowed to dangle from chair

3. Which of the following can be used to reduce wrist strain?
   a. Footrest
   b. Wrist rest
   c. Wired keyboard
   d. Wireless keyboard

Answer Key

| 1. | (a) | 2. | (d) | 3. | (b) |

Self-Practice Questions

1. What is the influence of a workstation design on symptoms pertaining to computer-related vision problems?
2. How can you work with the computer workstation environment to support the management of dry eye-related symptoms related to computer use?

CHAPTER 13

Sequential Management Considerations

Most patients complaining of symptoms of CVS are usually treated for dry eyes. In fact, they need two types of treatments:
- Restorative treatment
- Preventive treatment.

Restorative treatment involves a planned treatment regimen that requires some procedures and medications. It also involves the assistance of other specialties. The preventive side of the management falls into the realms of specialist practice. The objective is to minimize any disadvantage so that vision can be maximized and maintained. Vision is maximized by the use of lenses and vision is maintained by the use of lenses. A complete plan is essential for the total success that may be provided in sequential steps as shown in **Flowchart 13.1**.

INITIAL MANAGEMENT

The patient with symptoms of CVS visits the practitioner usually when he finds difficulties in visual performance. It means that the very first step is to correct any amount of uncorrected or under corrected refractive error of the patient reporting computer vision syndrome. There are reasons also. An uncorrected refractive error creates an additional demand on accommodative function. It may result in decompensated phoria. The results may be sensory fusion disturbances and blurred retinal images. Patient with uncorrected

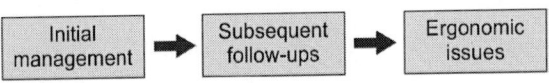

Flowchart 13.1: Sequential management consideration.

hyperopia has to accommodate to overcome his uncorrected hyperopia and he needs additional amount of accommodation to work on his computer workstation. Prolonged use of accommodation causes muscle fatigue which may result in accommodative symptoms. Uncorrected astigmatism results in visual symptoms and poor contrast sensitivity. Presbyopia is also an issue and care must be taken to correct it with a suitable correction for viewing distance of computer.

The correction of refractive error may be either in the form of spectacle lenses or contact lenses or LASIK surgery. Spectacles lenses are most preferred option to avoid contact lens-related complications that may occur because of inadequate blinking and wide open aperture and surgical complications of LASIK. Tinted lenses with antireflection coating may be the most suitable correction.

Together with the correction of uncorrected refractive error the patient needs to be explained about the complete treatment plan and their sequential steps. This is very important to ensure subsequent follow ups. The initial management may also include some eye-related exercise because exercise in general does create a feeling of well-being. The patient gets satisfaction that he made efforts and his efforts helped him treat the condition. Palming, visual scanning and frequent blinking are highly recommended procedures. They can be easily carried out while working on computers. The jobs like VDU create a situation where repetitive strain and restricted movement symptoms may crop up.

SUBSEQUENT FOLLOW UPS

On the subsequent follow up visit after the initial phase of treatment, if the patient still reports the symptoms of CVS, the another course of management may be added as shown in **Flowchart 13.2**.

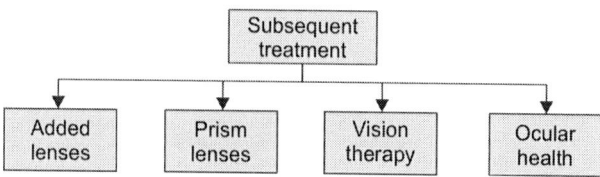

Flowchart 13.2: Subsequent treatment plan for CVS patients.

Added Lenses

Added lenses are very helpful in the treatment of symptoms related to CVS. They may be prescribed in the form of additional plus or additional minus over and above normal correction and may be added to the distance subjective refraction or to near or both to influence and affect binocularity. They may be prescribed either in single vision or bifocal form. Recently, Essilor have introduced specially designed lens for pre-presbyopic computer user, known as Anti-fatigue lens which has additional plus power at the bottom of +0.60D.

Minus lenses directly stimulate accommodation and secondarily convergence. Plus lenses relax accommodation and secondarily convergence. Plus lenses aid accommodation when deficient and help relax accommodation. Minus lenses are generally not used as it stimulates accommodation that may cause muscle spasm, fatigue, and eye strain. Added plus lenses are very helpful for patient with high AC/A ratio when esophoria is significant at near. Patient who report accommodative insufficiency and ill-sustained accommodation can frequently be treated with added lenses. Patients with accommodative excess are not benefitted by added lenses.

Prism Lenses

The long continuous work on VDU causes ocular fatigue that allows eyes to drift out and ocular posture changes to exophoric direction. The ultimate effect is loss of binocular single vision in the presence of motor imbalance. This creates an additional demand on fusional vergence function, indicating the need of prism lenses. When vertical and horizontal deviations are both present, the clinician should first consider prism correction for vertical component. As little as 0.5 diopter of vertical prism may be beneficial for fusion.

Vision Therapy

Vision therapy is the part of total optometric care and is a very scientific procedure to build up visual skills. One visual skill is built up on another. A significant number of patients with binocular vision and accommodative problems cannot be successfully treated with lenses and prisms or both. The lenses and prism prescription may be to increase the binocularity optically as long as they are on the eyes which can be then reinforced with vision therapy management.

Accommodative problem in which the difficulties is with relaxation of accommodation, vision therapy is the most suitable option.

Ocular Health

Poor tear film quality is the most common sign of patient complaining symptoms related to computer use which must be examined on the slit-lamp with different methods and a suitable treatment has to be prescribed in the form of lubricant eyedrop, ointments or gel together with eyelid hygiene.

ERGONOMIC ISSUES

Ergonomic issues are something which may be considered at the last as changing the working station or reorganizing the office environment may not be in the hands of the patient reporting symptoms related to computer use. The clinician may evaluate the working station by asking the patient to fill up the questionnaire form pertaining to working station evaluation and on the basis of the form; he may advise him certain remedial measures. The clinician may also discuss the ill-effects of poor ergonomics with the patient. An in detail discussion on visual angle, viewing distance, screen contrast, position of copyholders, footrest, armrest, chair and overall body posture may help the computer user to assume correct posture. The clinician may also inspect the office as a whole including furniture arrangement, lighting arrangement and overall postures of all employees and may make a report to submit the same to the concerned department so that a restructuring of the office ergonomic may be carried out to completely resolve the problem.

Multiple Choice Questions-Answers

1. **Which of the following will help reducing eyestrain when you work for long on computers?**
    a. Frequent blinking
    b. Shifting focus from near to far object
    c. Eliminating glare on screen
    d. All of the above

2. **Which of the following statements is not true?**
   a. Plus lens relaxes accommodation
   b. Minus lens relaxes accommodation
   c. Plus lens expands space and emphasizes ground
   d. Minus lens constricts space and emphasizes figure

3. **Which of the following statements regarding uncorrected refractive error is true?**
   a. Uncorrected refractive error may create additional demand on accommodation function
   b. Uncorrected refractive error may result in decompensated phoria
   c. Uncorrected refractive error results in poor contrast sensitivity
   d. All of the above

Answer Key

| 1. | (d) | 2. | (b) | 3. | (d) |

Self-Practice Questions

1. Mahesh, a 33-year-old stockbroker, presented with complaints of eyestrain and blurred vision after about an hour of online share trading. He had experienced these difficulties in the past also. The optometrist prescribed correction that did not work for him and hence he stopped using the same after about a month. He was otherwise healthy and was not taking any medications. Suggest management.

2. A 36-year-old software engineer with a single-vision hyperopic correction in his glasses is seeing well at distance but is having difficulty working on a VDU screen. Suggest the management.

3. What factors would you consider when deciding whether vision therapy is an appropriate treatment approach for computer-related vision problem?

4. What is the role of prism in the management of computer-related vision problem?

CHAPTER 14

Building up the Practice as a CVS Specialist

The load of patient's expectations is increased when they visit a specialist for consultancy and treatment. At least that is what I have realized over the period when I set up specialist optometry clinics. Building up a practice as a specialist requires setting up the goals and objectives of life and then making your way to achieve your desired goals. It is truly a daunting task yet so rewarding. Enthusiasm, commitment and a constant focus are more important than anything else. But once you establish and people start recognizing you as a specialist, a shift occurs and you are placed in a class that is much above common. This is only possible through hard work, passion and leaving no stone unturned approach.

A successful professional practitioner is master of his core clinical skills and is jack of all other skills. The professional skill per se is not sufficient for complete success. If you want success in your professional practice, you need to develop not only your core clinical skills but also some business and management skills of small business. This is more important when your practice is limited to a specialty. This is because a specialist practitioner works best on what he knows best and when taken away from his domain, he may not be as good. Nobody can deny the fact that the most successful practice needs to be delivered with highest quality clinical care. The other side is also a fact,i.e. if the practice is not been able to fetch patients, nobody would be benefitted with high quality clinical expertise. The bottom line is successful practice has to be delivered with high professional skills that is combined with business skills also. There are four common yardsticks to measure the success of the practice, they are shown in **Flowchart 14.1**.

Chapter 14: Building up the Practice as a CVS Specialist

Flowchart 14.1: Four yardsticks for success.

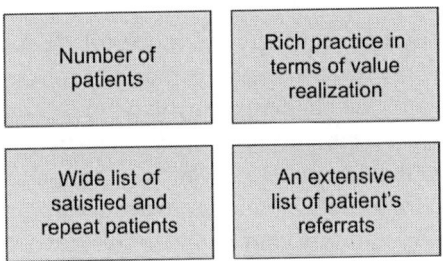

Flowchart 14.2: Eight simple ways to make positive attitude.

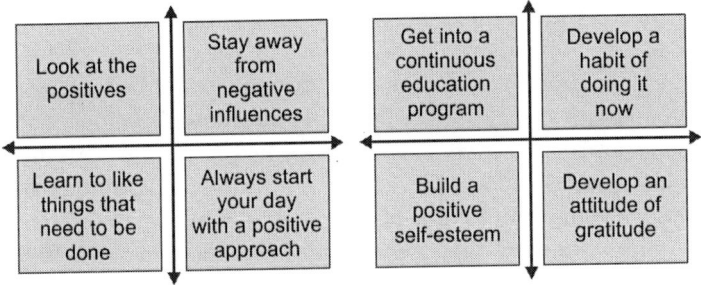

Your professional practice can be successful only when you take active role in creating and shaping your own practice. Only you can determine the type of practice you want to establish. Your attitude is the key to success. A man with positive attitude sees the invisible, feels the intangible and achieves the impossible. Positive attitude can be developed and there are eight simple ways to make your attitude positive as shown in **Flowchart 14.2**.

The following is the quick summary of the main areas on which the practitioner needs to work to build up a successful practice as a CVS specialist:

- Getting started
- Place planning to set up the practice
- Setting up the practice
- Promotions and marketing
- Practice management
- Stand proud and have self-commitment.

Chapter 14: Building up the Practice as a CVS Specialist

GETTING STARTED

When the doors are closed, everything behind the door appears to be lucrative. It is only when you start exploring a new opportunity; you come across with the challenges involved in it. I have had enough experience to set up specialty optometry practices and over the period I have realized that the only one way to set up a successful practice is 'sound preparation'. Preparations are needed at various fronts. You need to develop not only your clinical skills but also business and management skills of small business. When you make decision to venture out as CVS specialist, the first thing you need to do is to know your abilities and your interest. This is true for all kinds of specialist practice. If you are uncertain about your abilities, the best thing is to ask yourself one question, 'If you have to hire a CVS practitioner in your own clinic, what are the skills that you would be looking in an optometrist?' Once you get the answer note down your own skills on a paper and compare your own skills against them. The key is to make an informed decision. The reasons are simple. Bulk of the patients are seen young and middle age population who are associated with computer industry. They are well informed and educated. They will not accept anything less. Another way to be sure is to discuss with your professors about your strengths and weaknesses. This is how you would be able to develop a fair idea about the need for any training. In today's highly competitive world if you want to do something new and aim to excel in it, you must measure it. You will exactly come to know the true position, rather than just having a feeling. Then set up a bench mark. This is very important way to compare against the best in the peer group. If you cannot justify yourself on this ground, it implies there is scope for improvement. Believe me self-assessment is the best way to improve your own skill for the simple reason "it comes from your within". Your personal preferences are also important when you try to establish yourself as a CVS consultant. If you don't like the specialty, chances are you won't perform well in it. Therefore, it is important for you to figure out your personal preferences before it is too late.

Your clinical skills will make you expert in your chosen specialty, whereas your business skills will make you successful in the specialty. Business skill teaches you the art of goal setting and sharing your

Chapter 14: Building up the Practice as a CVS Specialist

goal with your team. It also teaches you to find out opportunities and how to capitalize on the opportunity. The business man can smell the opportunity and tries to make maximum out of it. The highly trained professional practitioner is exactly opposite. He is very good on his day-to-day job. But he cannot see the business opportunity and his entrepreneurship skills are based more on chances. An optometrist is a professional practitioner because he looks at the client as patient and puts his health concern ahead of selling a product or service. Treating patient is his profession, but the practice in which he delivers the professional service is a business. In fact, in order to be a successful CVS practitioner, he must be a successful business person. You need to look at yourself as 'Professional Business Person'. The point I would like to make is that the business man has tremendous work ethics. He runs the hard yards and lets everybody know the standards he expects. A great work ethics leads to a great team that guarantees success.

Management teaches the art of getting works done through people. Planning, directing, controlling and organizing are the four main principles of management. A successful practice is the result of the hard effort by a number of people who carry out their own set of responsibilities. Receptionist, assistant clinician, vision therapist and other office staffs form the complete team of a practice and a complete patient satisfaction can be only delivered if all work in harmony. Successful practice needs to be delivered with high quality clinical care which is combined with the management duties of small business **(Flowchart 14.3)**.

The last very important personal factor is your own dream. Don't overlook your dreams. They are a powerful incentive for you as you launch yourself as a CVS specialist. In fact, your dream lays the seeds of the beginning of romance with the specialty and your dream will only keep motivating you to continue with the romance. Knowing what you want is a critical first step to actually getting it. If you are very sure

Flowchart 14.3: Skills needed for success.

Clinical skills + Business skills + Management skills = Success assured about your dreams put it down on paper and justify it hundred times to make it more powerful.

PLACE PLANNING TO SET UP THE PRACTICE

The location and the size of the practice are two next most important areas. If you intend to have a "problem focused approach" you may not need a large space as only a few tests are to be applied. Comprehensive approach requires a series of tests to be done on each patient, to be followed by vision therapy, indicating the need for larger space. It is, therefore, wise to design a delivery model of your planned practice and then decide the size of the place. This is important to ensure that the design supports the function of the practice. In order to decide the suitable location, it is important to know the detailed demographic of the target population. A demographic survey is being conducted on the catchment area. CVS practice is normally most suited for urban areas where you can expect the patients from various computer and software companies. An urban area with nearness to IT industry or optical market is always more desirable. Many times practice may be opened within an existing optical shop or medical eye care office. This kind of symbiotic arrangement offers convenience to both patients and the business of practice. Sometimes, a location next to established ophthalmologist may provide strategic advantage and other time it may prove to be fatal. There are proven ways to look at this critical decision-making process. Analyze your core competence, put them in relation to your own strengths and weaknesses and see where you can capitalize. Once you are ready with this sort of analysis, it becomes easier for you to decide the most suitable location for your practice. Either you can go nearer to a strategic location or you can keep yourself away. The thumb rule is 'locate the practice within driving distance from the potential population, refrain from locations which are isolated from the main city'.

SETTING UP THE PRACTICE (FLOWCHART 14.4)

It is based upon the delivery model, get your fixtures and furniture, table tops, window and wall displays and have the entire infrastructure set up. Name your practice and make eye catching sign board. Professional interior designers can be hired to design and

Flowchart 14.4: Setting up the practice.

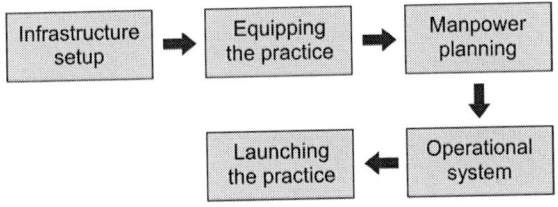

furnish the practice. Do not forget to allocate sufficient space for waiting. Make a list of the clinical equipments needed and order them. Some official equipment like office stationeries, computers, and printers are also needed. Once the infrastructural set up is complete, you need to recruit the man power and arrange their training to match your needs. When everything is set in its place, plan a suitable date to launch your practice. Circulate invitations to your family members, local authorities, local renowned personalities, eye doctors and others invitees. Launch may be with some events like introducing 'Optical Ollie,' or gifts to all guests. Advertise the event in local newspapers and on radio stations, and distribute fliers at local areas.

PROMOTIONS AND MARKETING

'Shoot for the moon, even if you miss, you will land up in stars.' To me this is the dynamic policy for planning the promotional strategy for your professional practice. Of course, high standard skills are needed, but if nobody knows about it, it is failure. Marketing of professional services starts with internal marketing and continues to extend with external marketing. External marketing communicates the intended message to potential patients to bring them to the practice whereas internal marketing establishes your credential when they visit your practice. The straight forward meaning is you need to be prepared. If your clinic does not look like what you are talking about or your practice does not signal what you intend to provide to your potential patients, you will lose credibility. Quite likely many people will take the impression that you send misleading messages. The bottom line is that there is a need for extensive planning in the promotional strategy as to the CVS specialist. There are two ends of marketing planning as shown in **Flowchart 14.5.**

Flowchart 14.5: Two plans for marketing your practice.

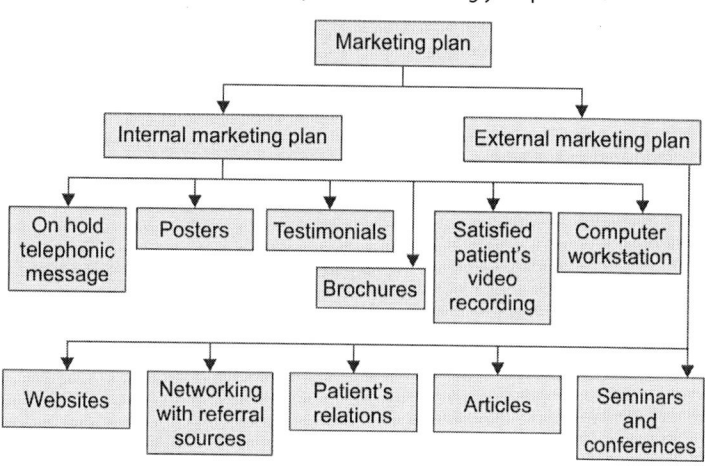

Internal Marketing

Internal marketing plan for professional services precedes the external marketing plan. Internal marketing prepares you to communicate with the external world. It also allows you an opportunity to check and correct your standing as purveyor of computer vision specialist. You need to analyze your position in the market place. You need to know how many other practitioners are there, how they practice, what their strengths are, who refers them, what is the current strength of the market and what is its future prospects. These are very important to decide the course of action in order to establish the practice profitably with high esteem. The plan also includes putting up posters on walls showing ill-effects of computer and poor ergonomics of computer workstation. Testimonials of satisfied patients and brochures on lenses designed for computer vision may be placed strategically. Another very small but extremely important idea is to run video recordings of satisfied patient's comments. Patient's comments are very powerful tools and if they are positive, can be used very effectively to motivate many others. A computer workstation may be set up somewhere near the waiting area with all attachments that would allow the patient to work on it for sometime, record his visual posture which could be later effectively used to explain the importance of ergonomics and bodily posture issues. Your practice would look like having computer friendly atmosphere. When the potential patient enters, he would take the impression that your office is geared to serve his needs. Most of the times this is sufficient to create which is very critical for any professional service to be successful.

External Marketing

Once you are through your internal marketing strategy, you can plan comprehensive marketing plan to announce to the world that you have something to offer computer users. One of the most valuable assets of a professional service is the network of referral sources that frequently send patients who need care. Building up the referral base is the key element of external marketing plan for professional practice. In general, total external marketing plan should include:
- Owning a website
- Networking with potential referral sources
- Building long-term relations with the patients
- Articles featuring practice and practitioner
- Workshop, seminars and conferences.

Owning a Website

The relevance of web is growing very fast. More and more people use the internet—not only as a source of information, but also as a platform for active exchange of experiences or to get advice on health issues. It implies that a web presence is more than just a necessity. Owning a personal website may be a good idea to make your presence known to the world at a very minimal cost. If you are not taking maximum advantage of web technology to market your professional services, you are behind the times, and missing out on huge opportunities. A website can attract new patients to your practice from across the street or far outside your local area. If your site has high rankings in the search engines under appropriate categories, you may get dozens of inquiries from people who otherwise would never hear about you. Participating in online discussion and message boards can allow you to network with a large group of people in your target market without leaving your practice. Appearing on live chats or webinars permits you to be a public speaker without the time and expense of travel. This also allows you to speak to national or global audiences. You can potentially attract larger number of prospects through social medias than with many more traditional methods of outreach. This may be very effective for people who have visual problems with computers as they are most of the time working on computers.

Networking with Potential Referral Sources

Today, if you really want to grow and survive in the professional practice, you need to maximize your chances of getting good referrals and developing a network of groups who refer you at regular interval. A CVS specialist may get referrals from ophthalmologists, other optometrists, satisfied patients, friends, relatives and other associates. Human resource manager of various software and computer companies may also be a great source of referrals for CVS patients. Asking for referrals requires that you have established credibility with the referral source and they have developed trust in you. So before you ask, spend time to deepen the relationship with the source. In the professional practice referrals do not happen by accident. They result from implementing, and then consistently monitoring, a well-organized business approach. Network building is very easy and effective if you execute the task to a dedicated person. The networking person should have a well-planned calendar to schedule contacts, mailing, follow up calls, workshop dates and other meetings. However, referrals can be only successful if you also have immediate feed backing system in place.

Building Long-term Relations with the Patients

Most health care issues are recurrent in nature and they are not a moment of crisis. They happen over a lifetime. This is especially true in case of patients having vision-related complains. Therefore, most effective practice should be ideally framed by long-term relationship. This is in the interest of both patient and the practitioner. The patient gets an honest and sincere treatment and the practitioner gets what exactly is the ultimate aim of his practice. In seeing the same patients again and again overtime, practitioners incrementally acquire considerable knowledge and that helps in managing subsequent problems. The relationship builds the loyalty and creates a network to get new referrals. You need to remember that long-term success largely depends upon the strength of relationship you share with your patients. Try and build up the practice on three C's as shown in **Flowchart 14.6.**

Flowchart 14.6: Three C's.

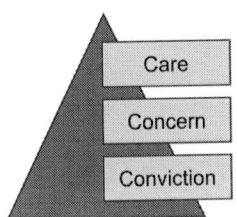

Articles Featuring Practice and Practitioner

Publishing a story or an article featuring the practice and the practitioner in a newspaper still works, especially for small newspaper or free circulation. There are magazines which are completely dedicated to computer industry, they may be a good source for potential patients. It is important that the story or the article you submit meets the high editorial standards for both contents and styles. Care should be taken that it does not sound promotional or self-serving. This may be considered as an ongoing process which does not have any cost to the practice. Probably, it may be a good image building exercise.

Workshops, Seminars and Conferences

Workshops, seminars and conferences are very effective media to promote you and your practice. A small group of people may be invited and a presentation may be delivered with some tea-coffee and snacks. This is very effective to influence a small group of people directly. Workshops are usually held during the evening and mostly on Saturdays. A seminar in a software company immediately exposes your practice to a large number of potential patients. At least, the person attending the event will be able to relate the signs and symptoms and then mouth publicity will pay additional dividends. During off-times, it may be adventurous ideas to conduct interprofessional workshops. Invite people from many professions and consider organizing joint workshops in which one from each of the profession presents the latest from his profession. This may be a good idea to reduce the cost or do the workshop at larger scale.

PRACTICE MANAGEMENT

Once all set in place, and people have started visiting your practice, you need an operational system in place. The profitability of your practice largely depends upon efficient execution of day-to-day operations and your ability to manage your own practice. A successful practice should have a complete professional approach where nothing is left to chances **(Flowchart 14.7)**.

There are certain basic rules for success. You must have full commitment towards your practice and your patients and you must assume all the responsibility to whatever you do or decide. All your actions should be planned and well-directed. You should be flexible in your opinion and open to other's suggestions. Your clinical practice should follow certain guideline. Develop a routine series of tests that you must do on all your patients. You must know to apply or avoid additional tests on suitable patients. Be thorough on your approach. Speakless and listen more while talking to your patients. Feel their pain and at the same time do not forget that you are into the business of professional practice. Always prescribe a suitable correction and provide options. Let your patient make choice. Educate the patient and monitor his condition. If needed, refer to an appropriate professional.

Always value yours and the patient's time. You must have system in place to handle appointment scheduling, cancellations and reappointments. Reminding the patients prior to their scheduled appointments works wonderfully. You need to take an important decision onto your professional fees that you would be charging to your patients. When you decide your professional fees, you must take several factors into consideration. Some of the important factors are your yearly revenue target, office overhead costs, your chair time cost, materials costs and other office expenses. Moreover, you also need to take into consideration how much other CVS specialists are charging in your region. You also need to decide on the fees structuring of vision therapy. Vision therapy fees may be charged based on per session or

Flowchart 14.7: Practice flow.

Practice flow → Appointment scheduling → Professional fees → Recording and analysis → Recalling and follow-ups as complete package for the planned treatment. A comprehensive recording system is very important. There are several exercises you need to do to make your practice successful. You must know your daily revenue, daily number of patient seen, sources of patients, staff performance, office overheads and other expenses. You need a comprehensive recording system so that you can do number crunching. At times you also need to check the patient's progress so that you may plan changes or otherwise. A comprehensive recording system would facilitate you to do all these exercise.

STAND PROUD AND HAVE SELF-COMMITMENT

As a clinician you garner all the respect of a medical practitioner from the patient and the society. You are always seen with eyes that are full of hopes. Sometimes because of professional expertise you also enjoy certain privilege. It implies that you must shoulder some extra responsibility. Your general attitude, ethical behavior and standard of practice should always be such that stand you out from others. More than this you must stand proud and have self-commitment. Patient notices your commitment. They will never accept anything which is not to their expectations. Top medical practitioners do not shy from consulting their fellow practitioner when they are not very sure. Remember more people fail not because they lack knowledge or talent but because they lack consistency, regularity and sincerity. Don't just keep your words, try and exceed it.

Well, I have long held belief that if you do not excel at a service. You are bound to invite failure. You need to invest your time and energy to educate and train yourself, your staff besides your investments in instrumentations and infrastructure to reap financial benefits from the practice. The success can never be the result of a chance. Recently, there has been a revolution in the eye care and eye wear industry. More complex and technologically driven products have been introduced. Personalization and customization of lenses are latest attraction. These changes in general are profoundly affecting the way the practice was done before and the way practice would be done now. Internet has also changed the way people now look at the any professional practice. Today's patient realizes that they have problem. They also know that they require solution. They do their own research as to the options available. Most often they also select one for them. The bottom line is that they are already aware of what the practitioner would advise them. Under such a typical scenario general approach to a specialist practice will not fetch success. Patient needs to be involved into the whole process to ensure predictable and repeatable results. The dynamics have changed and with the changed dynamics you need to change your approach.

Self-Practice Questions

1. What are the minimum set of test tools and instruments would you like to recommend to set up a computer vision syndrome clinic in private practice?

2. Explain how would you like to position your practice as a CVS specialist?

3. Explain how you would strategize to set up a strong referral program for promoting your practice as a CVS specialist.

CHAPTER 15

Vision Screening Program for Computer Users

Vision screening is a brief eye examination program that looks for potential vision problems and/or eye disorders. It does not aim to diagnose vision problems or an eye disorder. Vision screenings are often adopted by primary eye care providers or vision care institutes as a part of strategy to create awareness and also to promote the practice by reaching out to the desired section of population. If problems are recorded during a vision screening program, the subject is referred for complete diagnosis to be done in a clinical environment using sophisticated tests and equipment.

The increased use of computers in the workplace has brought about the development of a number of health concerns. Many individuals who work at a computer report a high level of job-related complaints and symptoms, including ocular discomfort, muscular strain, and stress. The level of discomfort appears to increase with the increase of computer use. The complex of eye and vision problems related to near work experienced during computer use has been termed "computer vision syndrome." Many individuals who work at a computer experience eye-related discomfort and/or visual problems. Vision screening program can help minimize such incidences associated with computer work and provide recommendations for preventing or minimizing their occurrence.

Studies have suggested that the majority of computer workers experience some common eye or vision symptoms. Most symptoms can be grouped under the following three broad categories for the purpose of designing an appropriate vision screening program:

1. Blur vision
2. Visual fatigue and stress
3. Dry eyes

The computer workers show typical difficulties with their vision. Usually, they do not complain of constant blurred vision unless there is a case of uncorrected or undercorrected refractive error. Intermittent blurred vision is the common complaint. The blurring occurring at irregular intervals at distance after near work is mostly the characteristic feature of an accommodative spasm or general accommodative dysfunction. This kind of blurred vision may be momentary when the person looks up from his near work or it may last for several hours after near work or in extreme cases it may carry to home causing difficulties at night. Intermittent blurred vision at near viewing distance may be because of dry eyes. The frequent color perception problems may be the result of poor display quality of the screen. Contrast and glare may also affect color perception temporarily. Blur vision is sometimes related to the inability of the eyes to steadily focus on a computer screen for a significant amount of time.

Visual fatigue and stress are common in computer users and are often associated with musculoskeletal discomfort. Workers who spend many hours on computers may report visual fatigue and discomfort related to their work environment as well as vision defects, psychosocial stress, and anxiety perception. Musculoskeletal discomforts in computer operators are due to non-ergonomic workstations and postural demands. The environmental factors, such as lighting, screen resolution and work arrangements, have also been suggested as causative factors for visual fatigue. They cause greater changes in visual function because of reduction in amplitude of accommodation. The increase in luminance has a negative effect on reaction time. Yellow-colored lights produce more visual fatigue compared to white lights. The presence of reflections causes confusion, with multiple attempts required to focus on computer screens and the need for additional accommodation responses. Working hours on computers without breaks can increase visual fatigue. Moreover, office work is sedentary and requires less physical energy than other jobs, but needs more mental attention and cognitive processes; sometimes constant work pressure can cause psychological stress. Visual fatigue is also individual related and is characterized by weakness of the eyes and general health condition. Eye fatigue appears because of the unconscious muscular effort of the eyes when preventive measures are not taken. The use of computers leads to a reduction in the amplitude of accommodation with an increase in exophoria. Close work also induces transient myopia, and it has been suggested that a temporary myopic shift may be a reliable objective assessment tool for computer-related visual fatigue.

Computer users commonly experience the symptoms of dry eyes. Dry eyes because of computer use are mostly attributed to evaporation of tears. There are several reasons why computer users are at a greater risk for experiencing dry eyes; they are decreased blink rate, higher viewing gaze angle, larger palpebral aperture, and lower workplace humidity.

The extent to which an individual may experience symptoms is largely dependent upon his/her visual abilities in relation to the visual demands of the task being performed. These vision problems are not new or unique to computer use. Many individuals in other highly visually demanding occupations also experience similar vision-related problems. However, the unique characteristics and high visual demands of computer work make many individuals susceptible to the development of eye and vision-related symptoms. Uncorrected vision conditions, poor computer design, and workplace ergonomics all contribute to the development of visual symptoms and complaints.

BATTERY OF VISION SCREEN TESTS

Vision screening program for people working on a computer should aim to diagnose a potential problem. The following tests may be included in vision screening battery:
- Computer vision syndrome (CVS) history
- High and low contrast acuity test
- Retinoscope
- Howell Phoria test
- RAF ruler test
- Dry eyes assessment

CVS History

History taking is one of the most important procedures of all health care examination and is equally important for vision screening program also. While it is important that the clinician himself takes the history from the patient for all clinical assessment, it may be collected through written questionnaire arranged in the most appropriate manner for the purpose of health screening as screening consists of identifying the presence of a disease or condition while it is in its preclinical stage. Computer Vision Syndrome (CVS) is a group of symptoms caused by continuous computer usages and could affect everybody who are active on using computers. A skillfully designed questionnaire for the purpose of taking history from people working on computers and complaining of one or more of symptoms of CVS can often help diagnose the condition, educate the subject to take precautionary measures before the worsening of the condition, and plan appropriate management. The author has designed the following CVS History Form (*see in next page*) for the purpose of screening of CVS patients.

High and Low Contrast Acuity

LogMAR charts are available in both high and low contrast for the purpose of visual acuity assessment. Low-contrast acuity test adds value to the overall vision assessment. Even if someone has 6/6 or 20/20 visual acuity, he may have eye or health conditions that may diminish his contrast sensitivity and make him feel that he is not seeing well. Deficiency of performance at low contrast can be significant, even if high contrast acuity is reasonably good. A significant difference between high and low contrast acuity may be symptoms of certain eye conditions such as cataract, glaucoma, or diabetic retinopathy.

Retinoscope

Retinoscopy is an objective method to determine the refractive status of the eye with respect to the point of fixation. The test is not dependent upon the subject's response. In screening, it is used to quickly measure long sightedness, short sightedness, astigmatism, or difference between two eyes—all of which could significantly reduce the visual performance. At the screening stage, it also helps to detect

CVS HISTORY SHEET

Name	
Age and gender	
Qualification	
Job Responsibilities	
Main Digital Gadget	Desktop/Laptop/Ipad
Leisure Time Activities	
Date of Assessment	

Please read the entire form and indicate the frequency and severity of the symptoms you experience during or after computer work. In addition, also provide your additional remarks with respect to each symptom, if you want to communicate as your own observation or perception. Please be specific and precise.	Rating			
Blurred Distance Vision				
Constant distant vision blurred or post work distant vision blurred or delay in focusing at distance after working for a longer period of time.	0	1	2	3
Additional Remarks:				
Blurred Near Vision				
Blur vision at close distance or blur vision while looking at computer screen or intermittent blurred vision at near-viewing distance.	0	1	2	3
Additional Remarks:				
Color Distortion				
Feeling as if there is a veiling effect on computer display and color perception is adversely affected.	0	1	2	3
Additional Remarks:				
Eyestrain				
Eyestrain or visual fatigue occurs when the eyes become tired because of intense use. Occasionally, it may be associated with ocular pain.	0	1	2	3
Additional Remarks:				
Dryness in eyes				
Feeling gritty or sand particles like sensation in the eyes, feeling blurred vision that improves on blinking, excessive watering of eyes.	0	1	2	3
Additional Remarks:				
Itching/Burning/Irritating eyes				
Feeling itching eyes/burning eyes, foreign body sensation and/or sore eyes. Often condition manifests in the form of excessive tears and excessive blinks.	0	1	2	3
Additional Remarks:				
Light Sensitivity				
Inability to tolerate bright light, you squint or close your eyes in bright light, and you feel more comfort working in dim light, lowering of chin while working, poor concentration.	0	1	2	3
Additional Remarks:				
Headaches				
Often feel headache towards the front of the head, occur most often towards the mid or end of the day. Occur in different pattern on weekends than during the week, sometimes it is more on one side of the head than the other	0	1	2	3
Additional Remarks:				
Neck/Shoulder/Backaches				
Feeling over exerted quickly, feeling numbness or stiffness around shoulder, neck and back	0	1	2	3
Additional Remarks:				
Wrist ache				
Difficulty in making a fist or gripping object, tingling sensation in hands, sudden sharp pain in hand, swelling or redness around wrist	0	1	2	3
Additional Remarks:				

Rating Scale		Any things else, if you want to communicate:
Never	0	
Occasionally	1	
Frequently	2	
Constantly	3	

the signs of pathology like cataract, keratic precipitates on the cornea, anterior synechia, keratoconus, etc.

Retinoscope can also be used to find out the accommodative response of the subject using one of the Dynamic Retinoscopy methods. A near target (MEM card) is attached to the retinoscope at patient working distance. With both eyes open and subject's distance correction in place, movement of reflex may be observed. If the movement is *with* add "plus lenses" and for *against* movement add "minus lenses" till the reflex neutralizes. If the final power is minus, the subject is over accommodating, indicating lead of accommodation. If the final power is in plus lens, the subject is under accommodating, indicating lag of accommodation. The normal range of accommodative response is +0.50DS to +0.75 Dsph.

Howell Phoria Test

Muscle balance can be measured using cover test at near and distance. But it is quite difficult to see any movement less than 3 diopters of prism and because the practitioner makes the estimate, this is essentially a subjective test. Howell Phoria Test is a more objective measure of muscle balance. It evaluates horizontal phorias at distance and near under more natural conditions than the cover test and Maddox Wing. The subject can see what is happening with his vision during the test. He can see that his performance is achieving a number and therefore immediately prompts a discussion on the relevance of the numbers. The practitioner will be able to relate the significance to the ability of the subject to resist visual fatigue. The diplopic image is created with six base-down prisms in front of the right eye. Moment by moment changes in the phoria can be measured. When the subject comes for full eye examination, he will already have several questions in his mind and will readily participate in the corrective measure.

RAF Ruler Test

RAF near-point rule is a routinely employed instrument in optometry practices to measure convergence amplitude, commonly known as near point of convergence (NPC), and accommodative amplitude, commonly known as near point of accommodation (NPA). The assessment of NPC is an important part of a routine eye examination as it serves as the primary assessment for the diagnosis of convergence insufficiency. Accommodative and convergence ability are two most important elements of binocular vision. RAF Rule provides a binocular gauge to measure convergence as well as accommodation. It consists of a 50 cm long rule with a slider holding a rotating four-sided cube. Each of the four sides has different accommodative targets with black prints on a white background which include:
- Side 1: A reduced Snellen chart
- Side 2: A section of the general post office telephone directory

- Side 3: Times Roman typeface
- Side 4: A dot on a line, the fixation target to assess NPC.

Dry Eye Assessment

Dry eye may be a primary concern of CVS since both a significantly reduced blink rate and increased corneal exposure have been observed during computer operation. The amount of time spent staring at a computer screen can worsen dry eye symptoms. While big-ticket devices are helpful, a thorough patient history is a vital first step toward dry eye screening and to describe how the condition affects the quality of life. An examiner can go into a detailed history with a questionnaire such as the Ocular Surface Disease Index (OSDI) or a Standardized Patient Evaluation of Eye Dryness (SPEED) to ascertain if the patient is symptomatic or not. These questionnaires are very efficient at discriminating between normal and dry eye subjects.

The tests as mentioned above are unique in the sense that they are not only able to measure aspects of visual performance but also demonstrate why these aspects of visual performance are important to computer users. During the screening process, we are not only trying to determine visual deficiency, but it is very important to relate this to the subject's understanding of their visual needs and why this might be a problem. The biggest travesty is the prevailing understanding that the refractive correction is the only treatment for all types of vision disorder. It is, therefore, important that the screening program also aim to propagate that there is more to vision than mere visual acuity.

Multiple Choice Questions-Answers

1. Which of the following is not the true objective of vision screening program?
    a. Look for a potential vision problem
    b. Diagnose a vision problem
    c. Create awareness
    d. Promote the practice by reaching out to a desired section of population

2. **Which of the following is not a symptom of wrist ache?**
   a. Difficulty in making fist
   b. Tingling sensation in hands
   c. Sudden pain in hand
   d. Feeling overexerted quickly

Answer Key

| 1. | (b) | 2. | (d) |

Self-Practice Question

1. Explain in detail the use and application of RAF Ruler.

Appendix

SPEED Questionnaire

Name: _____ , _____   **Date:** / /
          (Last)   (First)

DOB: / /   **Sex:** M / F

Report the type of **SYMPTOMS** you experience and when they occur:

Symptoms	At this visit		Within past 72 hours		Within past 3 months	
	Yes	No	Yes	No	Yes	No
Dryness, Grittiness or Scratchiness						
Soreness or Irritation						
Burning or Watering						
Eye Fatigue						

Report the **FREQUENCY** of the above-checked symptoms as never, sometimes, often or constant using the numbering system below:

Symptoms	0	1	2	3
Dryness, Grittiness or Scratchiness				
Soreness or Irritation				
Burning or Watering				
Eye Fatigue				

0 = Never, 1 = Sometimes, 2 = Often, 3 = Constant

Appendix

Report the **SEVERITY** of your Symptoms using the rating list below:

Symptoms	0	1	2	3	4
Dryness, Grittiness or Scratchiness					
Soreness or Irritation					
Burning or Watering					
Eye Fatigue					

0 = No problems
1 = Tolerable – not perfect but not uncomfortable
2 = Uncomfortable – irritating but does not interfere with my day
3 = Bothersome – irritating and interferes with my day
4 = Intolerable – unable to perform my daily tasks.

Do you use drops and/or ointment? _____

What drops do you use? _____

Bibliography

1. Applied Concepts in Vision Therapy. Leonard J Press.
2. Bhootra AK. Clinical Refraction Guide.
3. Bhootra AK. Ophthalmic lenses.
4. Bleything WB. Developing the Dynamic vision therapy Practice, published by Optometric Extension Program.
5. Carlson NB, Kurtz D. Clinical Procedure for Ocular Examination.
6. Claude GRONFIER The good blue and chronobiology: light and non-visual functions.
7. Cole BL. VDUs and Vision: Is the debate finished?
8. Duke – Elders Practice of Refraction, Revised by David Abrams.
9. Fannin TE, Grosvenor T. Clinical Optics.
10. Fundamentals of Computer, multimedia and internet by Aptech Limited.
11. Griffin JR, Grisham JD. Binocular Anomalies: Diagnosis and Vision Therapy.
12. Gunter K, von Noorden, Emilio CC. Binocular Vision and Ocular Motility.
13. Hanks A. What patients want?
14. Harrington S. "A protocol for the measurement of eye dominance in young children".
15. IACLE resource materials.
16. In Stewart D (Ed). System of Ophthalmology.
17. Khurana AK. Theory and Practice of Optics and Refraction.
18. Lavingia B. Computer Vision Syndrome.
19. Meriano C, Latella D. Occupational Therapy Interventions: Function and Occupations.
20. North RV. Work and the Eye.
21. Rucker F, Britton S, Spatcher M, Hanowsky S. Blue Light Protects Against Temporal Frequency Sensitive Refractive Changes. Invest Ophthalmol Vis Sci. 2015;56(10):6121-31. doi: 10.1167/iovs.15-17238. PMID: 26393671; PMCID: PMC4585532.
22. Scheiman M, Wick B. Clinical Management of Binocular Vision.

23. Sheedy J. Diagnosing and Managing Computer—Related vision problems.
24. Thierry VILLETTE Bad blue, good blue, eyes and vision
25. Video display terminal guidelines published by New Jersey State Department of Health and Senior Services.
26. Website references
    a. www.imiinnovations.com
    b. www.mdsupport.org
    c. www.prio.com
27. Zhao ZC, Zhou Y, Tan G, Li J. Research progress about the effect and prevention of blue light on eyes. Int J Ophthalmol. 2018; 11(12):1999-2003. doi: 10.18240/ijo.2018.12.20. PMID: 30588436; PMCID: PMC6288536.

Index

Page numbers followed by *f* refer to figure, *fc* refer to flowchart, and *t* refer to table.

A

Accommodation
 amount of 54, 54*t*
 amplitude of 57, 57*t*
 balanced range of 109
 function
  clinical examination of 56
  elements of 57*fc*
 lag of 60
 near point of 154
 negative relative 59
 positive relative 59
Accommodative anomalies 55*fc*
Accommodative excess 56
Accommodative facility 58
 testing of 58*f*
Accommodative function 52, 53
Accommodative insufficiency 56
Accommodative system 5, 7
Antireflection coated lenses, role of 98
Arms, pain in 19
Asthenopic symptoms 16
Astigmatism 45
Autorefractometry 40

B

Backaches 19
Bifocal lenses 114, 115*f*
Binocular accommodative
 facility 59
 range 59
Binocular balancing 48
Binocular vision 5, 7, 63
 clinical examination of 66
 function tests 67*fc*

Blinds 96*f*
Blink rate, decreased 84
Blinking 10*f*
Blue cut lenses, role of 100
Blue light, types of 103*f*
Blur vision 14*f*, 150
 at near, intermittent 14
Body posture issues 121*fc*
 related to 120
Body postures, incorrect 9*f*
Brock string 69*f*

C

Card test, hole in 38*f*
Clear near vision, plus lens to 108
Color perception 5, 8
Comfortable sitting posture 129*f*
Computer accessories 125*fc*
Computer and blink rate 10
Computer and body posture 8
Computer and presbyopia 111
Computer and vision 1
Computer display
 determinants 127*fc*
 issues related to 126
Computer monitor 125
Computer screen, letters displayed on 4*f*
Computer station 122*fc*
Computer use 82
Computer users, vision screen program for 149
Computer vision
 laws of 23, 25*fc*, 53, 94, 119
 syndrome 13, 31, 43, 149, 151, 152
 symptoms of 13*fc*, 28*fc*

Computer work, visual demands for 4
Computer worker
   fixates 25
   visual performance of 92
Computer workstation 88
   arrangement 119
Constant blurred vision 14
Contrast 5, 6, 128
   polarity 128
Convergence, near point of 70, 154
Copyholder 126
Cover test 68, 68f
Cross grid test 108, 109f
Cycloplegic refraction 45

D

Discomfort glare, solutions to 95
Dominant eye test 36
Dry eyes 82, 150
   assessment 151, 155
   causes 82fc
   diagnosis of 85
   disturb quality of life 83f
Duochrome test 48

E

Electromagnetic spectrum 101f
Ergonomic issues 134
Excessive head movement 78
Eye 2, 64
   accommodated 53f
   dryness, evaluation of 155
   larger opening of 85f
   movement 75, 117f
      disorder 75
      skills 77
      types of 75
   objective assessment of 38
   relaxed 53f
   sore 15f
   states of 53f
   tests for objective assessment of 39fc

F

Factors affecting computer workstation 120fc
Fixation 77
   disparity 68
Fixation distance 54
   different 54t
Four yardsticks for success 137fc
Furniture and fixture, issues related to 122
Fused cross cylinder test 60

G

General fatigue 21f
General symptoms 20
Glare 91
   disability 92
   discomfort 91
   effect of 18f, 92, 92fc
   presence of 94
   sequential management considerations for 95fc
   types of 91, 91fc

H

Hardware and attachment, issues related to 125
Head movement 117f
Headache 17f
High and low contrast acuity test 152
High energy visible blue 102
Howell phoria test 68, 151, 154
Hypermetropia 44

I

Ideal computer workstation 129
Ideal sitting posture 128
Illumination
   distribution of 98
   intensity of 98
   quality of 98
Itching eyes 15f

K

Keratometry 40
Keyboard 125

L

Lens
  added 133
  computer work with 112
  progressive addition 115, 117f
Lid aperture disorders 83
Light sensitivity symptoms 17
Logmar charts 152
Low blink rate 83
Low energy visible blue 102
Lower workplace humidity 85

M

Maddox rod test 68
Meibomian oil deficiency 83
Monitor angle 125
Monitor distance 125
Monitor height 125
Monitor size 125
Monitor with glare screen 93f
Mono vision 66f
Monocular accommodative facility 59
Monocular estimation method
  cards 61f
  retinoscopy 60
Mouse 126
Muscles
  inferior oblique 75
  inferior rectus 75
  lateral rectus 75
  medial rectus 75
  superior oblique 75
  superior rectus 75
Musculoskeletal symptoms 18
Myopia 45

N

Near addition
  determine 107
  tests for 108fc

Near duochrome test 109
Near-point world 1f
Nearsightedness 2
Near-vision lenses, occupational
    enhanced 116
Neck ache 19, 19f
Networking with potential referral
    sources 144

O

Ocular conditions, treatment of 89
Ocular gaze, higher 84f
Ocular health 134
Ocular motor dysfunction, clinical
    examination of 79
Ocular surface
  allergy 83
  disease index 155
Ocular symptoms 15
Oculomotor skills 5, 7
Overhead light source, glare from 93f

P

Palpebral aperture, larger 85
Patient counseling 88
Patient's visual environment 31
Phoria 67
Pinhole acuity 36
Pixel settings 127
Place while reading, frequent loss
    of 78
Poor comprehension 78
Poor eye teaming 2
Postwork distance blur 14
Practice flow 146fc
Practice management 146
Presbyope computer user, lens
    options for 114fc
Presbyopia 105, 106fc
  and computer use 105
  diagnosis of 106
Presbyopic patients, treating 112
Presence of reflection, checking 97
Preventive treatment 131
Prism lenses 133

R

RAF ruler test 151, 154
Reduced tear
 breakup time 83
 meniscus height 83
Refinements 48
Reflection and computer
 display 96
Refraction 98, 107
 subjective 46
Refractive error
 correction of 43, 46, 46fc
 types of 44
Refresh rate 128
Restorative treatment 131
Retinoscope 40, 151, 152

S

Saccades 77
Saccadic eye movement 80f
Schirmer's test 86, 86f
Screen color 128
Screen luminance 127
Sequential management
 consideration 131, 131fc
Setting up practice 140, 141fc
Short attention time 78
Shoulder pain 19
Single-vision lenses 114
Sjogren's syndrome 86
Skills needed for success
 139fc
Skipping lines 78
Slow reading speed 78
Smooth vergence test 70
Snellen test 50
Spherical endpoint 48

Step vergence test 70
Subsequent treatment plan 132fc

T

Tear
 breakup time test 87, 87f
 meniscus height 86
 thinning time 88
Torchlight examination 38
Trial and error method 110
Trifocal lens 115, 116f

V

Vergence facility test 71, 71f
Vergence range 70
Vision 2, 3
 process of 26fc
 screen tests, battery of 151
 suppressed 2
 therapy 133
Visual acuity 5
 test 35, 35fc
 with current correction 35
Visual fatigue and stress 150
Visual skills, primary 25
Visual symptoms 13
Visual system 2, 31
 control performance, elements
  of 25
von Graefe technique 68

W

Waist, pain in 19, 20f
Words, omission of 78
Workshops, seminars and
 conferences 145
Wrist pain 19, 19f